The Exceptional Potential of General Practice

The Exceptional Potential of General Practice

Making a Difference in Primary Care

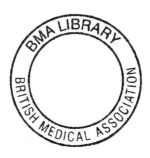

Edited by

Graham C. M. Watt

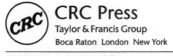

CRC Press

Taylor & Francis Group

Boca Raton London New York

CRC Press is an imprint of the
Taylor & Francis Group, an **informa** business

CRC Press
Taylor & Francis Group
6000 Broken Sound Parkway NW, Suite 300
Boca Raton, FL 33487-2742

© 2019 by Taylor & Francis Group, LLC
CRC Press is an imprint of Taylor & Francis Group, an Informa business

No claim to original U.S. Government works

Printed and bound by CPI Group (UK) Ltd, Croydon, CR0 4YY on acid-free paper

International Standard Book Number-13: 978-1-7852-3158-2 (Paperback)
978-1-1383-5368-8 (Hardback)

Visit the Taylor & Francis Web site at
http://www.taylorandfrancis.com

and the CRC Press Web site at
http://www.crcpress.com

Dedication

This book is dedicated to Julian Tudor Hart and Mary Hart, who blazed a trail for general practice at Glyncorrwg in South Wales and lit the way for others to follow.

If a man were permitted to make all the ballads, he need not care who should make the laws of a nation.

Andrew Fletcher of Saltoun (1653–1716), as inscribed on the wall of the Scottish Parliament.

The author was awarded the Saltire Society Fletcher of Saltoun Award for Science in 2018.

Contents

Acknowledgements

It has been a pleasure to compile this book. Colleagues cooperated splendidly, accepted quickly, wrote to order and responded positively to suggestions and queries. I hope I have done them justice.

Editorial responsibility has been mine alone, including the composition and order of the book, the examples chosen and the views expressed in linking text. None of the authors knew what others had written.

The *British Journal of General Practice*, the *Lancet* and the *British Medical Journal* have been very helpful in allowing previously published texts to be included. Colleagues at Taylor & Francis (Jo Kostner, Melissa Dalton, Linda Leggio, John Shannon) have also been very helpful in the final preparation and publication of the book.

I have had two major career influences. The first was the experience and example of working with Julian and Mary Hart at Glyncorrwg in South Wales. Having gone there in 1975 for my four-week medical student attachment in general practice at the University of Aberdeen, I was in no doubt that whatever career path in medicine I followed, it would involve some time working with them. Julian was not only talking and writing about the future, he was putting it into practice. Over 40 years later, the world of general practice has caught up with him in relation to population medicine, has forged ahead in terms of community practice, but is still in his wake on issues of accountability. At that time, it seemed a risk to go and work in the back of beyond, in a remote South Wales mining valley. On reflection, I never worked anywhere more central.

The second major influence has been the experience, pleasure and satisfaction of working with general practitioners at the Deep End, forging a productive academic-service partnership with expertise and respect on both sides. After 50 steering group meetings in eight years, all held in evenings after a busy working day, and well attended, it was clear that we were involved in something elemental about general practice. As a pre-institutional network of colleagues linked by passion and common cause, it was never less than a thrill to take part. It also gave me the confidence to write and compile this book.

The bridge between these two experiences was a career in academic general practice. With a background in epidemiology and public health, I was not a conventional candidate. I shall always be grateful to John Howie, Professor of

General Practice at the University of Edinburgh who encouraged and supported my application and to the late Sir William Kerr Fraser, Principal of the University of Glasgow, whose casting vote after a week's impasse gave me the Norie Miller chair in General Practice. That opened the door to 15 years as head of the department, which was a hugely productive and convivial time, as an academic generalist integrating teaching and research, helping to develop a new undergraduate curriculum, supporting the emergence of a dozen new professors, researching the Inverse Care Law and forging new links with service general practitioners.

As Tennyson put it, 'I am part of all that I have met' and a lot of it is in this book.

Graham C. M. Watt
University of Glasgow

Contributors

Harry Ahmed
General Practitioner and
    Clinical Research Fellow
Cardiff University
Cardiff, United Kingdom

Khairat Al Habbal
Clinical Instructor
Family Medicine and Social Medicine
Lebanese American University
Beirut, Lebanon

Breannon Babbel
Senior Public Health Program Manager
National Indian Health Board
Washington, DC

David Blane
Clinical Academic Fellow
and
Clinical GP Teacher
University of Glasgow
Glasgow, United Kingdom

Megan Blyth
General Practitioner
and
Clinical Academic Fellow
Cardiff University
Cardiff, United Kingdom

Kambiz Boomla
General Practitioner
Tower Hamlets, East London

and

Senior Lecturer
Centre for Primary Care and Public
    Health
Queen Margaret University London
London, United Kingdom

John Budd
General Practitioner
Edinburgh Access Practice
and
Co-ordinator of Lothian
Deprivation Interest Group
Edinburgh, United Kingdom

Peter Cawston
Full-Time GP Principal in a Deep End
    Practice
and
GP Cluster Quality Lead for Seven
    Deep End GP Practices in
    Drumchapel
Glasgow, United Kingdom

Amanda Connelly
General Practitioner
David Elder Medical Practice
Govan Health Centre
Glasgow, United Kingdom

Phil Cotton
Vice-Chancellor
University of Rwanda
Kigali, Rwanda

and

Professor of Learning and Teaching
University of Glasgow
Glasgow, United Kingdom

Vincent Cubaka
Family Physician, Senior Lecturer and
    Researcher
School of Medicine and Pharmacy
University of Rwanda
Kigali, Rwanda

Jan De Maeseneer
Retired Family Physician
Community Health Centre
    Botermarkt
Ledeberg, Belgium

and

Director
International Centre for Family
    Medicine and Primary Health Care
Ghent University, a WHO
    Collaborating Centre on PHC
Ghent, Belgium

James D. M. Douglas
General Practitioner
Tweeddale Medical Practice
Fort William, United Kingdom

Maria Duffy
General Practitioner
Pollok Health Centre
Glasgow, United Kingdom

Bridie Fitzpatrick
Research Developer/Manager
Scottish School of Primary Care
University of Glasgow
Glasgow, United Kingdom

Andrea Fox
Chief Medical Officer
Squirrel Hill Health Center
Pittsburgh, Pennsylvania

John Frey
Emeritus Professor
Family Medicine and Community
    Health
University of Wisconsin
Madison, Wisconsin

John Gillies
Retired Rural General Practitioner
Selkirk, United Kingdom

and

Deputy Director
Scottish School of Primary Care
Glasgow, United Kingdom

John Goldie
General Practitioner
Newhills Practice
Easterhouse Health Centre
Glasgow, United Kingdom

Iona Heath
Retired Inner City General
    Practitioner
and
Past President
UK Royal College of General
    Practitioners
London, United Kingdom

Sally Hull
General Practitioner
Tower Hamlets, East London

and

Reader
Centre for Primary Care and Public
   Health
Queen Margaret University
London, United Kingdom

Benjamin Jackson
General Practitioner
Conisbrough Group Practice
Doncaster, United Kingdom

and

Head of Teaching
Academic Unit of Primary Medical
   Care
University of Sheffield
Sheffield, United Kingdom

Tracey Johnson
Chief Executive Officer
Inala Primary Care
Brisbane, Queensland, Australia

Mark Kelvin
Director
Health and Social Care Alliance
   Scotland
Glasgow, United Kingdom

Andrew Lyon
Retired Converger
International Futures Forum
Aberdour, United Kingdom

and

Chair of the Deep End Steering
   Group, 2010–2016
Glasgow, United Kingdom

Becky Macfarlane
Speciality Doctor in Sexual and
   Reproductive Health
Sandyford Clinic
and
Sessional General Practitioner
Glasgow, United Kingdom

Ken McLean
Retired General Practitioner
Denny, Stirlingshire, United Kingdom

Stewart W. Mercer
Professor
Primary Care Research
and
Director
Scottish School of Primary Care
University of Glasgow
Glasgow, United Kingdom

Brian Milmore
General Practitioner
Govan Health Centre
and
Clinical Lead for Information in Govan
   SHIP
Glasgow, United Kingdom

John Montgomery
General Practitioner
and
Lead Clinician for Govan SHIP
Govan Health Centre
Glasgow, United Kingdom

Deborah Morrison
Portfolio General Practitioner,
   Combining General Practice in
   Glasgow, Research and a GP with
   Special Interest Post in Diabetes
Glasgow, United Kingdom

Anne Mullin
General Practitioner
Govan Health Centre
Glasgow, United Kingdom

Austin O'Carroll
General Practitioner
GMQ Primary Care Service for
    Homeless People
and
Programme Director North Dublin
    City GP Training
Dublin, Ireland

Patrick O'Donnell
General Practitioner
and
Clinical Fellow in Social Inclusion
Graduate Entry Medical School
University of Limerick
Limerick, Ireland

Tom O'Dowd
General Practitioner
and
Emeritus Professor of General
    Practice
Trinity College Dublin
Dublin, Ireland

Mona Osman
Instructor of Clinical Specialty
Department of Family Medicine
and
Co-Director
Refugee Health Program
Global Health Institute
American University of Beirut
Beirut, Lebanon

Euan Paterson
Retired Inner City General
    Practitioner
and
GP Palliative Care Facilitator,
    1999–2018
Glasgow, United Kingdom

Dominic Patterson
General Practitioner in Doncaster
and
Director of Postgraduate GP Education
Yorkshire and the Humber
    United Kingdom

John Patterson
Chief Clinical Officer and Deputy
    Accountable Officer
Oldham CCG
and
Medical Director
Hope Citadel Healthcare Community
    Interest Company
Oldham, United Kingdom

and

Co-Founder and Clinical Lead
Focused Care CIC
Manchester, United Kingdom

Tom Ratcliffe
General Practitioner
and
GP Trainer
and
Clinical Development Director
Modality Partnership
Airedale, Wharfedale and Craven
    Division
Yorkshire, United Kingdom

Douglas Rigg
General Practitioner
Keppoch Medical Practice
Possilpark Health and Care Centre
Glasgow, United Kingdom

Lisa Robins
General Practitioner Pioneer Scheme
    Fellow
Keppoch Medical Practice
Possilpark Health and Care Centre
Glasgow, United Kingdom

John Robson
General Practitioner
Tower Hamlets, East London

and

Reader
Centre for Primary Care and Public
    Health
Queen Margaret University
London, United Kingdom

Petra Sambale
GP Partner
and
GP Trainer
and
Lead GP Deep End Pioneer Scheme
Keppoch Medical Practice
Possilpark Health and Care Centre
Glasgow, United Kingdom

Jamie Sinclair
Building Connections Programme
    Manager
Supported by the Joseph Rowntree
    Foundation
Glasgow Centre for Population
    Health, the NHS, the Scottish
    Government and What Works
    Scotland
Glasgow, United Kingdom

Susan Smith
Professor of Primary Care Medicine
Royal College of Surgeons of
    Ireland
Medical School and General
    Practitioner
Inchicore Family Doctors
Dublin, Ireland

Sanjeev Sridharan
Director of the Evaluation Centre for
    Complex Health Interventions
Li Ka Shing Knowledge Institute
University of Toronto
Toronto, Ontario, Canada

Kenneth Thompson
Medical Director
Pennsylvania Psychiatric Leadership
    Council and Psychiatrist
Squirrel Hill Health Center
Pittsburgh, Pennsylvania

Kevin Thompson
Director
Academic Fellows Scheme
Division of Population Medicine
School of Medicine
Cardiff University
Cardiff, United Kingdom

Elizabeth Walton
General Practitioner
and
NIHR Clinical Lecturer
Whitehouse Surgery and The
    University of Sheffield
Sheffield, United Kingdom

Harry Hao-Xiang Wang
Associate Professor
School of Public Health
Sun Yat-Sen University
Guangzhou, PR China

and

Honorary Senior Lecturer
General Practice and Primary Care
University of Glasgow
Glasgow, United Kingdom

Graham C. M. Watt
Emeritus Professor
General Practice and Primary Care
University of Glasgow
Glasgow, United Kingdom

Suzanne Williams
General Practitioner
and
Director of Clinical Services
Inala Primary Care
Brisbane, Queensland, Australia

Andrea Williamson
General Practitioner
Homelessness and Addictions
and
Senior Clinical University Teacher
University of Glasgow Undergraduate
    Medical School
Glasgow, United Kingdom

Phil Wilson
Professor
Primary Care and Rural Health
University of Aberdeen
Aberdeen, United Kingdom

and

Professor
Child Health in Primary Care
University of Copenhagen
Copenhagen, Denmark

Introduction

This is a book for and largely by generalist clinicians working in the community plus others who wish to gain a better understanding of their work.

There are generalist services in hospitals such as accident and emergency (A&E) and geriatric medicine, and specialist services in the community such as mental health, child health and addiction treatments. The distinction between generalists and specialists is not about place or between primary and secondary care, but is about function. The function that this book addresses is the generalist clinical role in the community, which is called general practice in some countries and family medicine in others.

Health systems in different countries vary in their organisation, financial arrangements and underlying values. This book aims to transcend such differences by identifying common cause and shared practice among general practitioners working in different settings.

General practice has traditionally been seen and portrayed as the poor relation of specialist practice in hospitals. Most medical institutions, including the research and teaching to which medical students are exposed, are based on the dominant specialist paradigm.

We are at a turning point. As populations get older, multimorbidity accrues, resources tighten and health inequalities get wider, health systems and patients can no longer afford the fragmentation and inefficiency of multiple specialist services or rely on emergency care as the first point of call.

The balance between specialism and generalism needs to be reset, but power and resources are never redistributed by rhetoric alone. Examples and evidence are needed not just in individual practices but by large numbers of practices working together. To counter the dominance of specialism in health care, generalist clinical care needs a competing narrative based on solutions to the health care challenges of multimorbidity, fragmented care, increased pressure on emergency services and static inequalities in health.

No apology is made for concentrating on general practice in areas where lives are shorter, needs are greater and health care can make the biggest difference to patient's lives, combining specific treatments of known effectiveness with unconditional, personalised continuity of care. The challenge is to provide such care for all patients based on need. The 'unworried unwell' are not hard to reach but are easy to ignore and are often ignored. More than ever in the history of medicine, if health care is not at its best where it is needed most, inequalities in health will widen.

Although many examples in this book come from general practices in deprived areas, the challenges they address are common to generalist clinical care in most settings. The types of the problems presented by patients are familiar while their prevalence varies.

Fifty-four contributors from eleven countries range from general practitioners in the prime of their careers to those who can look back and reflect on four decades of work, while others are starting out. Some contributions are based on experience and values, while others draw on evidence-based practices with lists of references; however, all speak with authority.

The work of Julian Tudor Hart, to whom the book is dedicated and with whom several of the authors have worked, features strongly, not least because of the continued power of his writing.

This book draws on the past, by highlighting the pioneers of general practice in research, the population approach and advocacy; celebrates the present by featuring innovation, enterprise and passion in many settings; and looks to the future, not as a fixed destination, but as a common direction of travel with commitment to shared learning.

The major focus of the book is on practitioners who have made or who are making a difference to the development of general practice. This is a long march, spanning many individual careers. A single book can be neither definitive nor comprehensive in its coverage of examples, evidence and ideas. However, I hope this selection will be of interest to medical students, young doctors and experienced general practitioners, all seeking common cause in their profession.

> If we do not change direction, we shall arrive where we are heading.
>
> **Chinese proverb**

HOW TO READ THIS BOOK

Most of the individual contributions are short and self-contained. The list of contents may be likened to a tapas menu, therefore, and best sampled not in serial order but in several selections.

Chapter 1 summarises the exceptional potential of general practice under 12 headings, the first 6 of which are traditional while the second 6 look to the future.

The past

Chapter 3 describes the past, summarising the traditional and continuing strengths of generalist practice. Chapter 4 describes some early pioneers in research, population medicine and social advocacy.

The present

Chapter 9 describes five examples of community practice in Scotland, Ireland, Australia, the United States and Belgium, which have increased their local health system's capacity in different ways.

Chapter 13 provides international perspectives from countries at much earlier stages of primary care development. After listing the essential building blocks of a health care system and following Iona Heath's updated call for a general practitioner for every person in the world, the challenges in achieving this are described by colleagues from China, Lebanon and sub-Saharan Africa.

Chapter 6 describes the progress of general practitioners at the Deep End in the United Kingdom from its origin in Scotland to three other projects in Ireland, Yorkshire/Humber and Greater Manchester in England. Chapters 7 and 8 describe Deep End Projects in Scotland in more detail while Chapter 10 provides similar detail in the development of a learning health system in East London.

The future

Chapter 5 sets out challenges for the future, including multimorbidity, health inequalities, competition for power and resource and the need to recruit and retain general practitioners. In Chapter 2, Andrew Lyon argues that many of these challenges are not confined to health care but are symptomatic of general changes in society. How can practitioners 'be hospice workers for the old world and midwives for the new simultaneously?'

This is not a clinical book, but Chapters 11 and 12 cover challenges of special importance such as vulnerable children and families, people with mental health problems as a co-morbidity, palliative care and care for refugees and homeless people.

Chapter 16 describes cross-fertilising developments in education and training for general practitioners working in deprived areas, including how the Scottish GP Pioneer Scheme has built on the inspiring examples of the North Dublin City GP Training Scheme and the South Wales GP Academic Fellowship Scheme.

Chapter 14 examines different ways of producing evidence of change in both formal research studies and emergent development projects. In Chapter 15, Sanjeev Sridharan, taking the Deep End Project as a case study, reviews what needs to be learned from evaluation studies if colleagues in other places are to adopt and champion pioneering examples.

Finally

After a review of extra-curricular activities in Chapter 17, the book closes with a reflection in Chapter 18, a postscript on the philosophy of general practice in Chapter 19 and short biographies of the authors in Chapter 20.

1

The exceptional potential of general practice

In a 1953 essay on science and the modern world, the British mathematician and philosopher A. N. Whitehead wrote,

> The leading intellects lack balance. They see this set of circumstances, or that set, but not both sets together. The task of coordination is left to those who lack either the force or the character to succeed in some definite career. In short, the specialised functions of the community are performed better and more progressively, but the generalised function lacks vision. The progressiveness in detail only adds to the danger produced by the feebleness of coordination. We are left with no expansion of wisdom and with greater need for it. (1)

The thesis of this book is that generalism, far from being what's left for those 'lacking either the force or the character to succeed in some definite career', is a very definite career whose time has come but whose exceptional potential is still being realised.

CONSULTATIONS between practitioners and patients who are ill, distressed or who think they are ill are the cornerstone of practice, providing the starting points and turning points of care and involving decisions about the diagnosis and management of diseases from which almost everything else flows.

In 1979, Stott and Davis wrote a seminal paper entitled 'The exceptional potential in each primary care consultation', highlighting four components: the management of presenting problems, modification of help-seeking behaviour, management of continuing problems and opportunistic health promotion (2).

Consultations are the building blocks of care, but what needs to be built is a strong and comprehensive health care system. The challenge for clinical generalists is to show that general practices working together are a cost-effective way of improving population health and well-being, reducing fragmentation of care, stemming overuse of emergency services and reducing health inequalities.

The exceptional potential of general practice depends not only on consultations, but also on many other components of care.

CARING involves not only tuning in to patients' ideas, concerns and expectations, but also being ambitious for their health and health care. As Dr Francis Peabody once said, 'The secret of the care of the patient is in caring for the patient' (3). The 'unworried unwell', in particular, need a doctor who can use his or her greater knowledge and experience to anticipate and avoid problems. When a patient's health literacy, confidence and agency are low, self-help and self-management are destinations rather than starting points.

CONTINUITY of care via serial encounters helps to build the shared knowledge and confidence that lead to better outcomes. Julian Tudor Hart described his long-term relationship with a patient as 'initially face to face, eventually side by side' (4). For patients with complex problems and situations, seeing a familiar face avoids the time-consuming task of retelling their story to someone new. For practitioners, previous knowledge of and experience with patients means that more can be achieved within short consultations.

COORDINATION or orchestration of care involves bringing all relevant contacts, services and resources into play, with follow-up to assess the outcome.

Population COVERAGE requires universal access to care, a defined patient denominator, information systems that allow the measurement of omission and systematic measures to ensure high coverage rates.

Building CAPACITY requires adequate numbers of staff within the practice team, efficient deployment of their skills and strong working links with other services and resources, including embedded workers whenever possible.

COMMUNITY engagement involves establishing links with resources for health and health care in the community, including the third sector and voluntary groups. Link workers embedded within practices have been adept at developing this role.

CREATIVITY involves a constant search for better ways of doing things. Most local systems develop not from a blueprint or logic plan, but rather by trial and error, pursuing the positive and eliminating the negative.

COMMITMENT to the patients, practice and local community over a period of time provides the continuity and drive needed to overcome obstacles and achieve change.

CONSISTENCY implies that patients receive a similar standard of care wherever they access a general practice.

COLLEGIALITY involves common purpose, collective responsibility and the sharing of experience, views, information, evidence, activity and values so that the best anywhere becomes the standard everywhere.

CAMPAIGNING involves persistent advocacy with clear messages, examples and evidence of how health and health care can be improved.

REFERENCES

1. Whitehead AN. *Science and the Modern World*. Cambridge, UK: Cambridge University Press, 1953.
2. Stott NCH, Davis RH. The exceptional potential in each primary care consultation. *Journal of the Royal College of General Practitioners* 1979;29:201–205.
3. Peabody F. The care of the patient. *JAMA* 1927;88:877–882. doi:10.1001/jama.1927.02680380001001.
4. Hart JT. *A New Kind of Doctor*. London, UK: Merlin Press, 1988, 187.

Die when I may, I want it said of me
that I always plucked a thistle and planted a flower
where I thought a flower might grow.

Abraham Lincoln

2

Three horizons of general practice

ANDREW LYON

The twenty-first century finds us living through a period of change in our daily lives and the precepts by which we live. Such periods generally come along every 250 years or so.

Everything, including general practice, is affected by these changes. In the space of a relatively few years, the ideas that guide our efforts, the actions in which we are engaged, our view of the world, our health and our well-being – and all that goes with it – change beyond recognition. How are we to navigate these changes? The old is dying and the new cannot yet be born, causing morbid symptoms of system failure. How can we simultaneously be hospice workers for the dying regime and midwives for the new?" We are deep into the period of diminishing returns in almost all walks of life. Institutions and those who inhabit them are under almost unbearable pressure, and inertia in systems is a challenge in shifting to more sustainable policies and practices. Currently, three unhelpful 'isms' dominate (1):

Economism: Economy and profit are paramount.
Materialism: An excessive pursuit of fulfilment through material goods.
Individualism: Over-elevation of the individual as a primary unit of social
    organisation.

The pursuit of these 'isms' is widely embedded in global systems. Significant effort is engaged in identifying the extent of failure in essential systems – climate, food, water, energy, ecological diversity, and so on. There is much talk but insufficient action at the global or even national scale so far. We must learn to do something different.

In this short piece, I want to use the three horizons framework as developed by the International Futures Forum (2) to explore these questions based on my experience as the chair of GPs at the Deep End until 2016 (Section 6.1).

5

First Horizon: The first horizon (H1 in the chart below), is the here and now. In this horizon, the effort is concentrated upon addressing today's issues with today's best ideas and practices. Identifying, understanding, disseminating and improving current approaches are examples of such work.

Second Horizon: In the second, more medium term, horizon (H2), our current way of addressing challenges begins to feel less effective and no longer fit for purpose. Innovative approaches emerge, which hold the promise of more effective action. In H2, research and development functions and training help to realise the full power of new understanding for policy and action and have a key role to play alongside transitional actions, which begin to move us from existing to new frameworks.

Third Horizon: Simultaneously, in the third horizon (H3), innovations are taking place which often look fanciful to those working in the first horizon. It is from this horizon, based on fundamentally different premises, that radical innovation and completely new ways of doing things will emerge. Working in this horizon is more about the exploration of predicament, challenge, new thinking and different perspectives that keep possibilities for the future open.

Each horizon is present and relevant in every time frame Figure 2.1. It is the relationship between the perspectives which changes over time. The three horizons provide a framework not only for understanding but also for action and cooperation between perspectives that is relevant for action today and keeps options open for the future, which otherwise might be missing as new challenges emerge.

In general, a third horizon needs to be based on the principles different from the 'isms' outlined above, which means we are heading for system disruption.

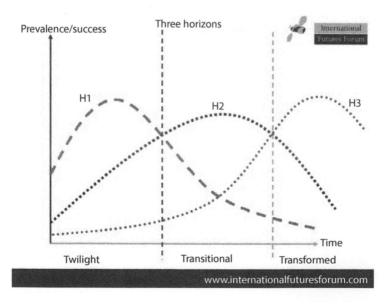

Figure 2.1 Three horizons (2).

GPs at the Deep End express their desired future – their third horizon – very clearly: a community-led general practice making a significant contribution to healthier, longer and fulfilling lives for those living at the Deep End.

Three kinds of actions might be taken now to move towards a more desirable future.

1. Action needed to address shortcomings in the system as it exists currently.
2. Actions that can be taken to bridge the gap between the current situation and that we want, including what we want to give up.
3. Actions, at small scale to begin with, which resonate with the future we want.

In taking action, ask:

- What can I do by myself as an individual GP?
- What can my practice do?
- What can the profession do?
- What must the professional work with others to do?

The future does not already exist. It is a place we are making and the making of it has the potential to change each of us, our relationships and where we are heading. The alternative is simply to accept that other people will make the future and we will all have to live in it. Which do you prefer?

REFERENCES

1. Hanlon P, Carlisle S, Hannah M, Lyon A. *The Future Public Health*, OUP, London, UK, 2012.
2. Sharpe B, Three horizons: The patterning of hope. www.international futuresforum.com.

Our rate of progress is such that an individual human being, of an ordinary length of life, will be called on to face novel situations which find no parallel in his past. The fixed person, for the fixed duties, who, in older societies was such a godsend, in the future will be a public danger.

A. N. Whitehead

3

Traditional strengths

This section describes some of the traditional strengths of general practice in the UK National Health Service, which since its introduction in 1948 has had the following basic features:

- General practitioners, either singly or more usually in partnerships, are contracted by the NHS to provide general medical and other services, mostly on a capitation basis with a fixed amount of funding per patient per annum, which is increased for some patient groups such as the elderly. A few procedures are paid for and incentivised on a fee-for-service basis.
- Treatment is free at the point of use and paid for via general taxation. Consultations with patients are largely devoid of financial considerations, which allows care to be inclusive and general practitioners to take an unconditional approach.
- Virtually, the whole of the general population is registered with a general practice with few gaps and very little duplication. Population coverage is achieved, therefore, by the sum of activity in a large number of clinical populations.
- General practitioners have a gatekeeping function whereby access to secondary care depends on referral by a general practitioner.

3.1 GATEKEEPING

Barbara Starfield is best known for showing that health systems with strong primary care achieve better outcomes at a lower cost (1). This longstanding observation predates most evidence-based medicine and associated clinical governance and quality initiatives. Although outcomes have undoubtedly improved more recently as a result of the mass delivery of effective interventions, the greater efficiency observed by Starfield was more likely a structural effect based on the activities of all practices, gatekeeping with and without gates.

Gatekeeping with a gate concerns access to non-emergency specialist care, whereby access to a specialist requires a referral by a generalist. Notwithstanding the occasional under- and over-referral of some patients, this arrangement generally results in more appropriate and efficient use of expensive investigations and treatments, compared with systems where patients have direct access to specialists.

Gatekeeping without a gate concerns access to emergency services such as out of hours, A&E or hospital admission. Here there is no gate, only a gateway that patients can go through at any time. When patients' problems are well managed in the community, they make less use of emergency services. The gateway is open but not used. If patients are dissatisfied with their care, cannot get access to care, or the complications of their conditions have not been prevented, they may flood through the gateway to access out of hours and accident and emergency services.

Health systems neglect gatekeeping at their peril. Small shifts in the balance of care between hospital and community (e.g. from 88% of care in the community and 12% in hospital to 86% in the community and 14% in hospital) are imperceptible in the community but can overwhelm hospital services. When generalist care in the community is weak, so that conditions are not ameliorated and their complications are not prevented, postponed or lessened, patients present for emergency care earlier than they should, with huge implications for the expense and sustainability of such services.

3.2 TOLERATING UNCERTAINTY

Clinical generalists provide patients with unconditional continuity of personalised care for whatever problem or combination of problems they may have. Generalists have to be able to diagnose and treat a wide variety of conditions, therefore, either separately in consultations with different patients or together within single consultations for patients with multimorbidity. However, clinical generalism is not only about diagnosis and treatment.

Sir James Mackenzie, a pioneer of general practice, wrote of his early clinical experience as a general practitioner in Burnley in north west England,

> I had not been long in the practice when I discovered how defective was my knowledge. I left college under the impression that every patient's condition could be diagnosed. For a long time I strove to make a diagnosis and assiduously studied my lectures and my textbooks without avail. For some years I thought that this inability to diagnose my patients' complaints was due to personal defects, but gradually, through consultations and other ways, I came to recognise that the kind of information I wanted did not exist .... (2)

Much generalist clinical care involves patients without clear diagnoses, with medically unexplained symptoms, whose management requires pragmatism, continuity and alertness to significant change. As Polynesia the Parrot in the *Dr Dolittle* books observed, '*a good doctor is a good noticer*' (3), sorting out the serious from the nuisance, not necessarily making a diagnosis, but using pattern recognition to spot when situations are unusual and require attention.

There is similar uncertainty with respect to treatment. Evidence-based medicine only goes so far. Despite their internal rigour, randomised controlled trials are often biased by systematic exclusion of complicated patients, practices and places.

In general, about a sixth of patients account for 50% of consultations in general practice. Multimorbidity is commonplace in this group of patients, but an exclusion criterion for many medical research studies. While evidence-based medicine may inform part of the management of such patients, it seldom informs the whole approach.

Alvan Feinstein, one of the founders of clinical epidemiology, concluded,

> Until the methods of science are made satisfactory for all the important distinctions of human phenomena, our best approach to many problems in therapy will be to rely on the judgements of thoughtful people who are familiar with the total realities of human ailments. (4)

The role of the clinical generalism is characterised, therefore, not only by the diagnosis and treatment of a wide range of conditions but also by the management of uncertainty in diagnosis and treatment and the need for pragmatic courses of action. In considering changes in skill mix in primary care, different types of health practitioners are likely to vary in their tolerance of uncertainty and their ability to manage this aspect of care without unnecessary investigation and referral.

> For medicine, being a compendium of the successive and contradictory mistakes of medical practitioners, when we summon the wisest of them to our aid, the chances are that we may be relying on a scientific truth, the error of which will be recognised in a few years time. So that to believe in medicine would be the height of folly if not to believe in it were not greater folly still, for in this mass of errors, there have emerged in the course of time many truths.
>
> **Marcel Proust**

3.3 KNOWING THE PATIENT

> It is often much more important to know what sort of a patient has a disease than what sort of a disease a patient has.
>
> **Sir William Osler (1)**

Cumulative knowledge of patients based on serial contacts is often an important component of generalist clinical care.

For example, symptoms or consulting behaviour that are unusual for an individual patient can be a warning sign, but this may only be apparent to a practitioner who knows the patient.

For patients with multiple long-term problems, meeting a doctor whom they know avoids the time consuming and the disheartening task of having to repeat their story for yet another time to a new person. For the doctor, previous experience and knowledge of the patient mean that more can be achieved within short consultations (Section 3.5).

Knowing the patient is one component of the CARE measure (Section 3.4), which was developed to ask patients whether the practitioner they had just seen was 'empathetic' (i.e. tuned in to their identity, history, circumstances and concerns etc). A study of over 3,000 general practice consultations showed that patients could report practitioner empathy without being enabled, but never reported enablement without practitioner empathy (2).

In the Care Plus Study (a randomised controlled trial including extended consultation time for complex patients in general practice – Section 3.4), it was impossible to agree on a definition of complexity to select suitable patients. Some patients with multiple conditions are not complex to deal with, while others with single problems can be very complex. It was not practical for researchers to collect sufficient information to make this distinction. Instead, patients were considered complex if their doctor thought they were complex, drawing on their cumulative knowledge and experience of patients (3). Doctors could not define complexity but knew it when they saw it. Looking later at the patients whom GPs had selected for the study, they were very complex, averaging five conditions each, but defining complexity had not been the starting point.

In the Govan SHIP Project (Section 7.1), general practitioners used their protected sessions and knowledge of patients to have extended consultations with selected patients whose complex problems needed full assessment, joint consideration with the patient and better care coordination (4).

These are only a few examples of the added value which comes from knowing the patients, their circumstances, personal history and how they cope with life's problems.

Such knowledge is unlikely to be acquired at medical school or early professional training and is accumulated slowly via experience in practice.

> To write prescriptions is easy, but to come to an understanding of people is hard.
>
> **Franz Kafka**
> *A Country Doctor*

3.4 CONSULTATIONS

STEWART W. MERCER

In our early work, the West of Scotland Enablement Study (1) focused on how the Inverse Care Law (Section 5.7) operates within consultations in deprived areas. We did this by collecting patient-completed questionnaires immediately after consultations. From 70 eligible practices approached, 26 GPs from 26 practices agreed to participate, giving an overall recruitment rate of 37% (36% in the high-deprivation group and 38% in the low-deprivation group). The participating practices and GPs did not differ significantly between high- and low-deprivation groups in terms of practice size, the age of GP or documented workload. A total of 3,044 patients completed the study questionnaire.

The patient response rate to the questionnaire was 70% (70% high-deprivation group, 71% low-deprivation group). Our first and very important finding, therefore, was that it was feasible to collect patient-reported measures on a representative sample of patients in deprived areas, with gold standard response rates. Our results showed that patients in deprived areas had more multimorbidity, more psychological problems, and more chronic health problems. Getting a consultation (access) took longer, and satisfaction with access was significantly lower in the most deprived areas. Patients in the most deprived areas had more problems (especially psychosocial problems) that they wanted to discuss in the consultation, yet the average consultation length was shorter compared with affluent areas. GP stress was higher and patient enablement was lower in encounters dealing with psychosocial problems in the most deprived areas. It was plain to see how the Inverse Care Law plays out in general practices in deprived areas.

The West of Scotland Enablement Study also confirmed the validity of a new tool we had developed, called the Consultation and Relational Empathy (CARE) Measure (2–4). This is a 10-item measure that captures the patients' views on GP empathy. In a secondary analysis of the study, we made the simple but important finding that patient enablement requires GP empathy (5). GP empathy does not guarantee patient enablement (because many factors influence enablement that are out with the consultation), but enablement never occurs with low empathy. In the current era of self-management support, this is a crucially important message.

In the subsequent work, we developed and tested the CARE Approach as an online toolkit, and as a book (6,7), to help GPs and other practitioners improve their empathy in the clinical encounter. The CARE Measure is now widely used throughout the world, having been validated in a range of countries and languages.

This quantitative research on general practice in the Deep End was supported by a qualitative study of patients' views on primary care (8). Data were gathered through 11 focus groups involving 72 patients. The two broad themes which emerged were firstly, patients' views of their GPs' competence and secondly, their perception of the GP's empathy or 'caring'. Views on competence were often based on whether patients had 'successful' outcomes with that doctor in the past. 'Caring' related to being listened to by the doctor, being valued as an individual, the doctor understanding 'the bigger picture' and explanations that were clear and understandable.

It was clear from this work that patients from deprived areas sought GPs who understood the realities of life in these areas, and whom they could trust as both competent and genuinely caring. Without this, patients judged the GPs as socially distant and emotionally detached. Continuity, relational empathy and enough time in consultations were the key factors in achieving this.

Having established how the Inverse Care Law operated, we investigated the benefit of changing one aspect of this in the Keppoch practice in Possilpark, the most deprived practice in Scotland. The Keppoch Study investigated the benefit of extended consultation lengths for patients with complex needs (9). We measured GP stress and patient enablement in 300 consultations before the introduction of extended consultations and in 324 consultations at follow-up after one year.

Again, response rates of 70% were obtained. This was only possible in this extremely deprived population by having a full-time researcher based in the practice, who was able to administer the questionnaire face to face with patients. We found that GP stress was higher in complex consultations at baseline. Consultation length in complex consultations was increased on average by 2.5 minutes by the intervention. GP stress decreased in the consultations after the introduction of extended consultations and patient enablement increased. GPs' views in qualitative interviews supported the findings, with the GPs reporting that more anticipatory and coordinated care was possible in the extended consultations.

Our next major step was the Living Well with Multimorbidity programme of research, funded by the Scottish Government Chief Scientist Office from 2009 to 2014. This was a £800,000 programme of work to develop a primary care-based complex intervention for patients with multimorbidity in deprived areas. This was done hand in glove with Deep End GPs and nurses in a co-production approach. We initially gathered practitioners' views on managing patients with multimorbidity in Deep End practices, which they described as an 'endless struggle' (10). We gathered patients' views on how multimorbidity affected their everyday lives (11) and examined the epidemiology of multimorbidity in a large, nationally representative data (12) set to help establish our target group for the intervention.

We showed that multimorbidity had a devastating effect on the quality of life of younger patients in deprived areas (13) and was associated with huge increases in unplanned hospital admissions, especially when linked with deprivation and mental health problems (14). Less than 10% of patients in Scotland had four or more physical health conditions, but they accounted for one-third of unplanned and almost one-half of potentially preventable unplanned admissions to hospital. Compared to those living in the most affluent areas with no long-term conditions and no mental health problems, patients living in the most deprived areas with four or more conditions and a mental health problem were 51 times more likely to be admitted to hospital for a potentially avoidable unplanned admission (14).

We then developed, piloted and optimised the complex intervention which we called CARE Plus (15). The intervention was co-designed by the research team with GPs, nurses, and patients working and living in very deprived areas. The intervention consisted of much longer consultations (up to 40 minutes) for targeted multimorbid patients with continuity of care, an empathic approach and self-management support aimed at enabling patients. The GPs and nurses also received training and support. Finally, we tested the feasibility of CARE Plus in an exploratory cluster RCT in Deep End practices (16). This allowed flexibility in how the intervention was organised and delivered in different practices while retaining the core 'active ingredients'. We showed that it was feasible to recruit practices and patients to the RCT and to retain them in the study, achieving follow-up rates at 12 months of almost 90% in both the control and intervention groups (gold standard rates, due to the hard work and persistence of our research team – Section 14.1). We showed that CARE Plus was likely to be effective in maintaining the quality of life and was very cost effective, coming well below the UK government's threshold for introducing a new treatment (16).

Recent work includes an early evaluation of the Deep End Link Worker Project (see Chapter 8), in which Deep End practices were randomised either to receiving a link worker and practice funding for staff well-being or to usual care (17). The evaluation combined qualitative with quantitative measures. The intervention worked well in terms of staff well-being in practices that fully integrated the approach but less well in those who did not. Patients appreciated the links approach, and those who engaged with the link workers and the suggested community resources showed meaningful improvements in mental health (see Section 11.4). Overall, quality of life was not improved, but the time span of the evaluation was short (nine months of follow-up from baseline). High-quality research on social prescribing is lacking internationally, and we have recommended more research on this before wide-scale adoption (18).

3.5 CARING

> There is only one rule of practice.
> Put yourself in the patient's place.
>
> **Joseph Lister**

*I shadowed a GP working in one of the most deprived areas of Glasgow. She arrived at 7.20 am on a Monday morning to deal with 38 items of correspondence, all needing to be checked and prescriptions altered, a patient phoned, or arrangements made, before the day even started. The telephone calls to patients all began the same way: 'This is Dr xxxxx, Hello John, Hello Helen etc'.

As the on-call doctor on a busier day than usual, she completed seven house visits that morning, each taking 30 minutes. It took an hour to enter all the details back in the practice and make the necessary arrangements, leaving five minutes for lunch. A colleague who took over the on-call for the afternoon made three more home visits, dealt with 22 telephone consultations and then held six emergency appointments.

The afternoon surgery ran for three hours and would have lasted longer if all the booked patients had attended. Problems addressed included cancer, depression, agoraphobia, asthma, self-harm, bereavement, domestic violence, heart failure, alcohol abuse, dementia, social neglect and so on, often in combination. She left for home after a 12-hour day, with 61 items of correspondence still to deal with.

I did not see any short or trivial consultations. There were no 'worried well' patients, but a worried doctor leaving no loose ends when dealing with a series of patients with complicated health issues and other problems, all of whom she

* This essay was published previously in the *British Journal of General Practice*. Watt G. Discretion is the better part of general practice. *Br J Gen Pract* 2015. doi:10.3399/bjgp15X685357.

knew well. One patient said 'Dr xxxxx' is the only person I can relate to'. Another came in grim-faced, avoiding eye contact, almost in tears, but left 15 minutes later, beaming a smile.

I was struck by the intensity of the day, every patient getting the same attention. The doctor was too busy to put on an act: 'We have to focus on every single patient and listen. A lot feel they bother us and we cannot fob them off by being stressed or not dedicating time'. The practice has learned from experience that it is unsafe to assume that if problems are serious, patients will consult in time.

There are three GP partners and none work full-time: 'You cannot work fully concentrated for a whole day without recovery time'. The practice is wondering whether it might attract more students to their list to dilute the clinical load. Burnout is an ever-present hazard. The level of work is hard to sustain.

The consultations I observed showed a GP at the top of her game. The previous contact, shared knowledge and trust were fundamental to what could be achieved in a short space of time. Despite the pressures of practice in a deprived area (1), the GP was ambitious for what she could achieve with, and for, her patients.

One seldom gets the opportunity to observe a GP through a whole working day. What I saw in Glasgow reminded me of working with Julian Tudor Hart at Glyncorrwg in South Wales. He is best known for research on high blood pressure, but his daily practice and long-term achievements were characterised by his unconditional approach to all patients, whom he came to know well, whatever problems or combinations of problems they had. In the BBC documentary series on NHS Pioneers, Mary Hart said, 'Many people sentimentalise us, but we were just doing our job, for which we were paid, providing the NHS for our patients' (2).

In an article with Paul Dieppe, Tudor Hart described the poisonous effects which can arise when, for whatever reason, health professionals become indifferent to what happens to the patient in front of them (3). I remember him talking about the importance of finding something to like about every patient. There was no one about whom there was not something to like.

In the 1950s, Collings described poorly resourced areas of general practice as 'sufficient to turn a good doctor into a bad doctor in a short period of time' (4). Such gross effects are less common today. A more subtle effect is whether practitioners set the bar high or low when dealing with patients.

The incentives of the Quality and Outcomes Framework, involving only 12% of GP consultations (5), have little to do with this aspect of practice. Professionalism and caring for patients are what matter, and both are at the discretion of individual practitioners.

Consultation rates are often used as crude measures of practice activity and proxy indicators of health need. Such data convey nothing of the duration, content, quality, or consequences of consultations, and their use in resource allocation formulae sustains the Inverse Care Law (6). What I saw in one day in one practice in one part of the country goes unrecorded in the scheme of things, reflects poorly on the NHS commitment to equitable resource distribution, but spoke volumes for the professionalism of one GP.

3.6 CONTINUITY

*Everyone is familiar with Aesop's fable of the tortoise and the hare. Although the hare was faster over short distances, it was the plodding tortoise which won the race.

The recent history of policies and initiatives to address inequalities in health is littered with hare-brained schemes, exchanging long-term effect for short-term display. Many of these schemes are conceived in mad March, when there is the end of year money to spend. Like genetically programmed crops, they disappear when the year is out.

Deep End GPs describe the life cycle of many community initiatives which, by the time they get established and become useful, are already starting to wind down. In maintaining a list of local community resources, the continuing challenge is to keep up to date.

Health check programmes are often in vogue and can process large numbers of people through the initial stages of risk assessment, but when most of the resource goes into the beginning of the process, such programmes often fizzle out.

A frequent notion of initiatives to address health inequalities is the 'transformative encounter', in which patient behaviour is changed by a single professional intervention. But such examples, however celebrated, are notable for their rarity, and unlike the reality of working with the large numbers of patients with multiple morbidities and complicated social problems.

Patients with long-term problems have few consultations in which diagnoses are made, but dozens and sometimes hundreds, in which the business of the consultation is living better with risks and conditions and avoiding or delaying their complications. Yet the focus of most medical education, evidence, guidelines and NHS policies to address inequalities is at the start of this journey.

In the film *Brief Encounter*, Trevor Howard plays a GP who has a series of short and intense emotional encounters with Celia Johnson in Carnforth railway station. Young people watching this film today are prone to say, 'Not a great deal happened'. The same is often true of brief encounters in primary care.

Serial encounters in general practice are a fact, and individual patients attend all of them. The encounters may or may not feature continuity, in terms of practitioner contact or information sharing. They may or may not involve cumulative learning, co-production (with the patient taking an increasingly active role) or the building of social capital, by which patients acquire increasing knowledge, contacts, experience and confidence. But in the absence of adequate time to get to the bottom of problems, sustained effort and effective links with other professions and services, few of these things are likely to happen. Instead of serial progress, there are cycles of repetitive, non-productive behaviour.

* This essay was published previously in the *British Journal of General Practice*. Watt G. The tortoise and the hare. *Br J Gen Pract* 2011. doi:10.3399/bjgp11X601415.

Such trajectories are seldom simple. They stop and start, with reverses, delays, diversions and the intrusion of events. There is no 'logic plan'. But within this Brownian motion, there can be a constant purpose and steady progress – the tortoise rather than the hare.

In his book, *A New Kind of Doctor*, Julian Tudor Hart described 25 years of care of a big muscular man, who had been invalided out of the steel industry following an industrial accident (1).

> For the staff at our health centre it was a steady unglamorous slog through a total of 310 consultations. For me it was about 41 hours of work with the patient, initially face to face, gradually shifting to side by side. Professionally, the most satisfying and exciting things have been the events that have not happened: no strokes, no coronary heart attacks, no complications of diabetes, no kidney failure with dialysis or transplant. This is the real stuff of primary medical care.

In a spat with Tudor Hart, Professor David Sackett, a pioneer of clinical epidemiology and evidence-based medicine, remarked that it was the first time he had been likened to a snail. Ironically, it was by the snail-like progress that Tudor Hart improved the health of his practice population (2).

The future challenge is not to re-create Tudor Hart's pioneering example of anticipatory care, but to deliver its essential elements via local health systems with general practice at the hub. Key ingredients are flexibility, constancy and an always open door. Perseverance is more important than pace. Nor is perseverance one long journey; it is many short journeys, one after another. A recent systematic review revealed that increased continuity of care by doctors is associated with lower mortality rates (3).

Great things do not just happen by impulse but are a succession of small things linked together.

Vincent Van Gogh

The disappearance of personal doctors is greatly exaggerated. At a recent meeting of three Deep End GPs (Chapter 6) with a journalist, there were over 60 years of local experience in the room, and an enormous amount of knowledge, commitment and compassion on display. Such knowledge is no longer the preserve of GPs and is frequently acquired by other members of the health team. Exchanging such knowledge is an important team function.

All that GPs can do to reduce inequalities in health is via the sum of the care they provide for all their patients. To realise this contribution, the NHS needs not only to address the Inverse Care Law, increasing the volume and quality of care where needs are greatest, but also to understand, value and support serial encounters in primary care.

BOX 3.6: Publishing in your domain

Sometime after the above article was published, the author received an unsolicited email from Article Delivery Services, offering updates on 'who is publishing in your domain.' The titles of the sample articles included:

- Radial-arm-maze behaviour of the red-footed tortoise
- Ancient colonisation and within-island vicariance revealed by mitochondrial DNA phylogeography of the mountain hare (Lepus timidus) in Hokkaido, Japan
- The occurrence and dynamics of polychlorinated hydrocarbons in brown hare (Lepus europaeus) in southwestern Slovakia
- The dazed and confused identity of Agassiz's land tortoise, Gopherus agassizii with the description of a new species and its consequences for conservation
- Picture–object recognition in the tortoise Chelonoidis carbonaria
- Comparison of S(+)- ketamine and ketamine, with medetomidine, for field anaesthesia in the European brown hare (Lepus europaeus)
- The hare (Lepus granatensis) as a potential sylviatic reservoir of Leishmania infantum in Spain
- Rhabdomyosarcoma in a terrestrial tortoise (Geochelone nigra) in Nigeria: a case report
- Comparison of intraosseous and peripheral venous fluid dynamics in the desert tortoise (Gopherus agassizii)
- Species boundaries and host range of tortoise mites (Uropodoidea) phoretic on bark beetles (Scolytinae), using morphometric and molecular markers
- Sulawesi tortoise adenovirus-1 in two impressed tortoises (Manouria impressa) and a Burmese star tortoise (Geochelone platynota)
- Variation in growth and potentially associated health status in Hermann's and spur-thighed tortoise (Testudo hermanni and Testudo graeca)

Subsequently, the author received repeated invitations to submit his upcoming work to the *Integrative Journal of Veterinary Sciences*.

3.7 COORDINATION

As multimorbidity has become a commonplace, partnerships and teams have developed and the number of referral services has increased, coordination has become an important feature of generalist clinical practice.

Hector Berlioz, the French composer, was a coordinator par excellence, and there are lessons in his autobiography for general practitioners (1). Forced into medical studies by his father, who was a doctor, he stuck it for two years before finding refuge and the beginning of a new career in the Musical Conservatoire of Paris.

Although best known now as a composer, based on such works as his *Symphonie Fantastique*, the choral piece *La Damnation de Faust* and opera *Les Troyens*, Berlioz was famous in his time as an orchestral conductor. This led to invitations all over Europe.

Berlioz records that while the concert superstars of the time, such as Pagannini on the violin and Liszt on the piano, could turn up at the last minute to enthral an audience, his job as a conductor was much more complicated. Arriving several days ahead of the concert, the first task was to assess the players in the local orchestra. As the composer of many of the pieces to be played, he knew the music inside out, but whether and how a piece could be played depended on the types of instrument which were available and the talents of the instrument players. If an instrument was weak or absent, he would re-orchestrate the piece to be played by others.

There was other work to do, such as teaching the parts, getting the orchestra to play together and transforming their rough first attempts into a polished final performance, the whole becoming something more than the sum of its parts. Then he would repeat all this at his next destination.

His example applies readily to the coordination of medical care. Similar to a composer, the practitioner has a clear idea of the care that is required, but whether it is delivered depends on how the available talents and resources are orchestrated. Finally, the care has to be conducted and the final test is in the performance.

As composers, orchestrators and conductors of care, practitioners determine whether and how coordinated care is delivered. As an audience judges a performance, patients and their carers judge the quality of coordinated care.*

3.8 COVERAGE

Back in the 1960s, before rubella immunisation and the Abortion Act, a sixth (unwanted) pregnancy in a 42-year-old Glyncorrwg woman resulted in a child with severe brain damage. The mother had had no apparent illness, but there had been an epidemic of rubella in our village during the first weeks of her pregnancy. The whole family was affected: the father's smoking and alcohol problems went out of control into diabetes and coronary heart disease. As the child grew he became unmanageable, with all ground floor

---

* Berlioz also pioneered mass participation. His requiem mass was scored for an orchestra of 450 players, 'or multiples thereof'. But that is another story.

windows smashed and replaced by cardboard. The home became a cave. In the insensitive jargon of health economists he became a high consumer of services, first diagnostically, later for social educational support, now (as his exhausted relatives die or capitulate) for the most costly service of all, full-time residential care.

So, when rubella immunisation became possible, we wanted it to succeed. At that time secondary school absence was running at 20% in 13-year-olds at the local comprehensive, and at least this proportion was therefore presumably not immunised. I wrote to our local medical officer asking for a list of girls missed, so that we could get them immunised. 'I can give you the names of the ones we did,' he wrote back, 'but how can I know the ones we didn't?'

With this anecdote, Julian Tudor Hart began his classic paper in the *British Medical Journal* on 'The measurement of omission' (1). By comparing the numerator of what he had done with the denominator of eligible patients, he described the 'rule of halves' whereby about a half of the patients had a blood pressure measurement, half of those with high blood pressure were on treatment and half of those on treatment had their blood pressure controlled. Treatment of high blood pressure had been effective, but only an eighth of the eligible patients got the benefit of treatment. Similar results were found for diabetes and other long-term conditions.

The Rule of Halves reflects the natural entropy within poorly organised systems of human behaviour whereby things tend not to be done, or are done badly, so that patients continually leak out of the system. The relevant statistics are simple, where D represents the denominator of eligible patients and N represents the numerator of activity.

N/D = the coverage rate
D-N generates a list of patients who have not been included

The first task in addressing the rule of halves is to screen patient records, not patients, to establish what has not been done. Records are then flagged to alert the practitioner to attend to the task when the patient visits next. In this way, coverage is increased cumulatively, as part of routine work without the need for special measures. The two preconditions of this approach are that patients' presenting concerns are dealt with first and that there are sufficient time and resource to include additional tasks.

The approach of case finding, as described above, contrasts with screening whereby special arrangements are made to contact the patient population, usually at a time and place chosen by the screener. When special equipment is involved (e.g. mammography), or coverage is required quickly (e.g. flu vaccination) this approach is necessary, but for ongoing ascertainment and management of risks in general practice, case-finding is more efficient.

Clinical researchers consider that they have done well if they achieve 70% participation rates. General practice has no such luxury. In the UK Quality and Outcomes Framework, the majority of incentivised clinical targets required 90% coverage rates.

It is something of a paradox that while public health professionals tend to have little contact with the public, health professionals with significant public contact tend not to think about public health. Few health professionals in general practice would consider themselves to be epidemiologists, but primary care teams have by far the largest experience of converting denominators into numerators on a continuing basis and dealing with all sorts of people to achieve that effect.

3.9 CLINICAL GENERALISM IN SCOTLAND

JOHN GILLIES

Keeping the NHS and the patient happy are sometimes two completely different things.

This quote from GP Dr Euan Paterson (Section 11.5) comes from a meeting held during the Essence of General Practice Project (1) and illustrates the tension that is inherent in general practice between ensuring that we meet external NHS measures of quality and performance, like the Quality and Outcomes Framework (QOF), while still meeting the needs of our patients. Essence was published in 2009 and QOF has since been abolished in Scotland though not in the rest of the United Kingdom, but this tension has not gone away.

How does this relate to generalism? Generalism was seen by GPs as a key role for the future in Essence. Reeve's subsequent definition of generalism is both succinct and comprehensive (2).

Practice which is person, not disease-centred, continuous, not episodic, integrates biotechnical and biographical perspectives, views health as a resource for living well, not as an end in itself.

If we relate Reeve's definition to the problem that Paterson sets out, it is clear that, at least in theory, generalism is the answer. It embraces a focus on the individual, not just the disease. It suggests that continuity, with its implicit focus on relationship-based care, is important. This is reinforced by an explicit need to look not just at biotechnical aspects of care, but also biographical aspects – the patients' social history, family, community, cultural norms and expectations. Finally, it is founded on a non-Utopian conception of health. This is vital in the world of general practice, where GPs meet every day with children, women and men with chronic conditions that can be helped but not always cured. Helping them meet their goals in living active and flourishing lives (3), rather than focussing on achieving biomedical or biochemical perfection, is central to generalism and good general practice.

Scotland has a distinguished history of the development of general practice in the fields of undergraduate and postgraduate education, quality improvement and academic excellence (4,5). Iona Heath (Section 13.2) relates these achievements to high literacy rates in Scotland since the 1770s (due to John Knox's insistence that everyone should be able to read the Bible) followed by the Scottish Enlightenment. She suggests that these are important historical factors in creating a climate for the flourishing of general practice. Certainly, some key features of the Enlightenment – allowing people to think for themselves, a climate of tolerance of dissenting views, and perhaps most importantly, a belief that the world can be improved through rational thought and action, are prerequisites for any discipline that, like ours, has both scientific and relational elements.

Since devolution in 1999, the NHS in Scotland has gradually diverged from its counterpart in England. Organisational change, amounting to churn, has been rapid and bewildering in England. Policies that promote market forces and the appearance of large corporate players like Virgin in general practice have not happened in Scotland. This is partly due to legislative change and also a cross-party consensus that it is undesirable. In Scotland, the past five years have seen significant legislation to enable integration of health and social care, and in 2018, the first Scotland-only GP contract.

The context within which GPs practice in Scotland has significant differences from the rest of the United Kingdom. Scotland has the most remote populations in the United Kingdom as well as many populated islands. It also has some of the most deprived populations, concentrated in Greater Glasgow but also in Edinburgh, Dundee and Ayrshire. Generalists have to adapt to the people and communities they serve. Rural generalists may need skills in pre-hospital immediate care, palliative care and community hospital work, and may have a commitment to 24-hour urgent care. Those who work in the Deep End need to be able to deal every day with overwhelming patient demand and the health and social consequences of poor housing, intergenerational poverty, and drugs and alcohol (6).

You can trace the beginnings of generalism in Scotland back to the Dewar report. In 1912, this report, informed by the evidence of a committee which travelled widely through the highlands and islands and, unusually included a woman, highlighted the dire poverty of the people and the desperately poor state of provision of medical services. The resulting Highlands and Islands Medical Service (HIMS), financially supported by the State, served as a blueprint for the NHS in 1948 (7).

Generalism in 1912 was not the same as generalism in 2018, of course. However, accounts of the commitment of HIMS doctors to their patients show clearly that these were not doctors who limited their practice to the biotechnical and were often much involved in community engagement and public health (Section 4.3).

Dewar is still actively remembered and discussed in Scotland by the RCGP and other bodies, including a significant conference on the centenary of the publication of Dewar in 2012 (8). While the Deep End movement has allowed a focus on the grossly reduced life expectancy and healthy life expectancy in deprived areas (9), as well as the needs of GPs and their teams working under great pressure, remote areas require an excess cost of supply due to population sparsity and difficult geography. Deep End practices still labour under the Inverse Care Law of Tudor Hart, an abiding feature of the NHS today (10).

However, there are major changes underway which have the potential to strengthen generalism in Scotland in the future. Two Chief Medical Officer reports introducing and explaining 'realistic medicine' (11,12) have the following principles:

- Moving towards shared decision making
- Building a personalised approach to care
- Reducing harm and waste
- Reducing unnecessary variation in practice and outcomes
- Managing risk better
- Becoming improvers and innovators

All of these relate well to a generalist approach, but particularly the first two. Indeed, an early response to the publication of the first report was by GPs suggesting that these principles represented what they had spent their professional lives attempting to do, sometimes in the face of contractual and system disincentives.

However, enabling realistic medicine will require realistic research to provide an evidence base for generalist approaches. An outline for how this might work is provided by the Scottish School of Primary Care (13). Close collaboration between service and academics, carefully chosen research questions and innovative designs could provide 'middle ground' practice and policy research within a much shorter timeframe than standard RCTs. This would also, of course, require a novel research support stream.

In addition, the new GMS contract for Scottish GPs (14) moves away from the disease-centred approach of the QOF to one based on clusters of general practices working together, both to develop and implement quality within practices and to engage and influence the new integrated joint boards. Behind the new contract lies the premise, central to Essence, that 'contracts should enable rather than limit developments in general practice.' There is much potential there to be realised.

Scotland has advantages of scale over England. Being small (in population if not geography) means that relationships between parts of the now integrated health and social care system—Scottish Government, integrated joint boards, NHS Education in Scotland (NES), Health Improvement Scotland (HIS), Royal College of General Practitioners (RCGP), British Medical Association (BMA), primary care academics, and others – can, with skill and care, be developed to the advantage of health professionals, patients and communities. This offers the opportunity for generalism to flourish in the future. It is an opportunity that we must not waste if we are to start addressing Euan Paterson's important conundrum.

3.10 39 YEARS IN PRACTICE

JAMES D. M. DOUGLAS

3.10.1 Practice reflections

I have worked with my current GP partners for 34, 25, 20 and 2 years. My manager and reception team also have decades of experience with me. These trusting team relationships between ourselves, our patients and our wider team add value to patient care and our professional endeavour. We feel safe with innovation and take pride in the collective micro-developments and front-line delivery projects that have advanced local health care but also sustained our team's self-worth.

Postgraduate and undergraduate education have been a core practice value. A total of 90 people have given us youthful medical enthusiasm in exchange for holism and communication skills.

Over the decades, I have observed the whole of medicine adopting the GP educational ethos and communication skills. This has fundamentally improved the patient experience in the United Kingdom and been driven by GP trainers, the RCGP and GMC.

I am currently a pilot GP tutor for the first UK undergraduate longitudinal integrated clerkship in medicine. Students spend the whole of their fourth year at medical school in general practice. It is medical education turbo charged, using the tool of general practice to 'teach medicine, rather than general practice'. The longitudinal clerkship method will secure the future not only of general practice but also of the NHS.

In 2005, postgraduate medical education implemented Modernizing Medical Careers and GP Specialist Training. GPST gave us status, structure and educational governance; however, with rigid frameworks, we lost the joy of experiential learning. On balance, GPST has been an improvement for patient safety and professional standards.

I gained international friends and insights with WONCA (World Organization of Family Doctors) Rural. It is very affirming to share the lived experience of general practice at an international conference workshop. It made me appreciate how fortunate we are in UK general practice where quality improvement and patient safety cultures are world leading.

New diseases, drugs and technologies have changed and challenged practice. The battle between microbes and humans has been fascinating over decades. We get clever with technology; they get clever by mutation. They can still deliver that fatal punch at any age.

The close relationship with families over decades and generations is the strength of UK general practice. When you have seen the child in utero exposed to cigarettes, drugs and poor diet grow into a damaged teenager who repeats the cycle, you are observing epigenetics in action.

My younger observations on health inequalities have been explained by new science including epigenetics and shortened telomeres which describe premature aging.

Mental health has been revolutionised over my 39 years. The prevalences of Autism and ADHD have increased profoundly, but I can only speculate why. We understand emotionally damaged young people and learning disabilities much better now as psychiatry has advanced. We now take suicide very seriously. societal attitudes to mental health have been revolutionised by social media, but social media also generate mental health problems.

Thirty-five years ago, my practice became an early adopter of computers. They have been our most powerful tool but remain fundamentally flawed as we try to capture the human condition in binary code.

I used to attend deliveries, go to road accidents and attend life-threatening medical emergencies. We have had to cede these roles to specialist nurses and paramedics but gained confidence in multimorbidity and chronic disease management. The individual complexity per patient has developed exponentially.

Cancer care and end-of-life care have been revolutionised by medical technology.

Patient continuity delivers quality, but is now a precious intervention which needs to be managed and 'prescribed' as an actively managed process for groups of patients who will benefit including learning disability, palliative care and challenging younger adults.

The new challenges of 'overdiagnosis' and 'overtreatment' have emerged in my final GP years. They require a fundamental rethink of medicine's future role in society, with new primary care teams lead by expert medical generalist GPs.

3.10.2 Personal reflections

I was inspired by my undergraduate tutor to choose general practice. My other passions during university studies were scuba diving and marine science. I aspired 'to be a GP on the West Coast of Scotland with an interest in Diving Medicine'.

After 39 years, the breadth and depth of clinical general practice remain fresh. I enjoy undergraduate teaching and I am kept curious by researching Lyme disease.

The small rural town of Fort William has given me work–life balance. The beauty of the place and the outdoor sports made it difficult to leave. On several occasions, I could have moved into academic general practice or occupational medicine, but I made an active decision to stay and develop my career in one place for family stability. My wife worked with me as a community nurse and gave me new insights on our patients.

Our greatest achievement has been our family and their children. Two of our children are artists and two are doctors.

I recall a 'gulp moment' at the start of my career as a GP partner. Can I do this for decades, in the same place, with the same people? Many professionals see their careers in seven-year segments and move on. However, the decades spent in one community have given me social and professional capital which have made me more effective and efficient.

In my first decade, the Underwater Training Centre gave me an early opportunity to teach professional divers Diving Medicine and treat 'the bends'. I published cases, new methods of treatment and research. It was exciting to go into hyperbaric chambers to treat divers and at other times fly in helicopters as a member of the Lochaber Mountain Rescue Team.

I love the generalism of general practice but also developed special interests. Those special interests have come, gone and come back again. Occupational Medicine came in my forties with an MD describing a new cause of Occupational Asthma in salmon processing (Section 4.1). The big advantage of rural communities is the easy visibility of new diseases and industries. Research that threatened new jobs needed social and professional capital to complete. I worked with factory engineers and immunologists to prevent asthma.

I then developed my research skills further with GP publications on flu vaccinations and flu PCR diagnosis. Then came a new theme of rural health. I ran a big NHS project on rural education and policy. I dropped occupational health and research but importantly remained a clinical GP.

Lyme disease was described in the year I graduated. Twenty-three years ago, I published an unusual Lyme case report and I am now describing a local epidemic. The ecosystem of the ticks is in my garden, so it is easy to understand zoonotic transmission in my patients. I feel privileged to be involved in advancing medical science by understanding the ecology of humans and microbes at the end of my career as a GP. The scientific uncertainties keep me on my toes in my efforts to do the best for my patients.

I am certain that none of this would have happened if I had not 'kept the day job' as a GP in one rural community. Rural visibility, personal curiosity and self-confidence have made it happen. It is interesting that our children are creative. On reflection, a lot of my work has been about being creative in general practice.

REFERENCES

3.1 Gatekeeping

1. Starfield B. Is primary care essential? *Lancet* 1994;344:1129–1133.
2. Mair A. *Sir James Mackenzie, M.D. 1853–1925 General Practitioner.* Churchill Livingstone, Edinburgh, UK, 1973, p. 47.
3. Lofting H. *Dr Dolittle.* Jonathan Cape, London, UK, 1922.
4. Feinstein AR. The need for humanised science in evaluating medication. *Lancet* 1972;300:421–423.

3.3 Knowing the patient

1. Osler W. *Aequanimitas with Other Addresses.* HK Lewis, London, UK, 1946.
2. Mercer SW, Jani B, Wong SY, Watt GCM. Patient enablement requires physician empathy: A cross-sectional study of general practice consultations in areas of high and low socioeconomic deprivation in Scotland. *BMC Family Practice* 2012;13:6.
3. Mercer SW, Fitzpatrick B, Guthrie B, Fenwick E, Grieve E, Lawson K, Boyer N et al., The Care Plus study – A whole system intervention to improve quality of life of primary care patients with multimorbidity in areas of high socioeconomic deprivation: Cluster randomised controlled trial. *BMC Medicine* 2016;14:88.
4. General Practitioners at the Deep End. Deep End Report 29: GP use of additional time as part of the SHIP Project. www.gla.ac.uk/deepend.

3.4 Consultations

1. Mercer SW, Watt GCM. The Inverse Care Law: Clinical primary care encounters in deprived and affluent areas of Scotland. *Annals of Family Medicine* 2007;5:503–510.

2. Mercer SW, Reynolds W. Empathy and quality of care. *BJGP* 2002;52(Supplement):S9–S12.
3. Mercer SW, Watt GCM, Maxwell M, Heaney DH. The development and preliminary validation of the Consultation and Relational Empathy (CARE) Measure: An empathy-based consultation process measure. *Family Practice* 2004;21:699–705.
4. Mercer SW, McConnachie A, Maxwell M, Heaney DH, Watt GCM. Relevance and performance of the Consultation and Relational Empathy (CARE) measure in general practice. *Family Practice* 2005;22:328–334.
5. Mercer SW, Jani B, Wong SY, Watt GCM. Patient enablement requires physician empathy: A cross-sectional study of general practice consultations in areas of high and low socioeconomic deprivation in Scotland. *BMC Family Practice* 2012;13:6.
6. Bikker AP, Cotton P, Mercer SW. *Embracing Empathy in Healthcare. A Universal Approach to Person-Centred, Empathic Healthcare Encounters.* Radcliffe, London, UK, 2014.
7. Fitzgerald N, Heywood S, Bikker AP, Mercer SW. Enhancing empathy in healthcare: Mixed-methods evaluation of a pilot project implementing the CARE Approach in primary and community care settings in Scotland. *Journal of Compassionate Healthcare* 2014;1:6.
8. Mercer SW, Cawston PG, Bikker AP. Patients' views on consultation quality in primary care in an area of high deprivation; a qualitative study. *BMC Family Medicine* 2007;8:22.
9. Mercer SW, Fitzpatrick B, Gourlay G, Vojt G, McConnachie A, Watt GCM. More time for complex consultations in a high deprivation practice is associated with increased patient enablement. *BJGP* 2007;57:960–966.
10. O'Brien R, Wyke S, Guthrie B, Watt G, Mercer SW An 'endless struggle': A qualitative study of GPs' and Practice Nurses' experiences of managing multimorbidity in socio-economically deprived areas of Scotland. *Chronic Illness* 2011;7:45–59.
11. O'Brien, R., Wyke, S., Watt, G., Guthrie, B., Mercer, SW. The 'everyday work' of living with multimorbidity in socio-economically deprived areas of Scotland. *Journal of Comorbidity* 2014;9:62.
12. Barnett B, Mercer SW, Norbury M, Watt G, Wyke S, Guthrie B. The epidemiology of multimorbidity in a large cross-sectional dataset: Implications for health care, research and medical education. *Lancet* 2012;380:37–43.
13. Lawson KD, Mercer SW, Wyke S, Grieve E, Guthrie B, Watt GCM, Fenwick EAE. Double trouble: The impact of multimorbidity and deprivation on preference-weighted health related quality of life a cross sectional analysis of the Scottish Health Survey. *International Journal for Equity in Health* 2013;12:67. doi:10.1186/1475-9276-12-67.
14. Payne R, Abel G, Guthrie B, Mercer SW. The impact of physical multimorbidity, mental health conditions and socioeconomic deprivation on unplanned admissions to hospital: A retrospective cohort study. *CMAJ* 2013;185:E221–E228. doi:10.1503/cmaj.121349.

15. Mercer SW, O'Brien R, Fitzpatrick B, Higgins M, Guthrie B, Watt G, Wyke S. The development and optimisation of a primary care-based whole system complex intervention (CARE Plus) for patients with multimorbidity living in areas of high socioeconomic deprivation. *Chronic Illness* 2016;12:165–181.

16. Mercer SW, Fitzpatrick B, Guthrie B, Fenwick E, Grieve E, Lawson K, Boyer N et al., The Care Plus study- a whole system intervention to improve quality of life of primary care patients with multimorbidity in areas of high socioeconomic deprivation: Cluster randomised controlled trial. *BMC Medicine* 2016;14:88.

17. Mercer SW, Fitzpatrick B, Grant L, Rui Chng N, O'Donnell CA, Mackenzie M, McConnachie A, Bakhshi A, Wyke S. The Glasgow 'Deep End' Links Worker Study: Protocol of a quasi-experimental evaluation of a social prescribing complex intervention for patients with multiple complex needs in areas of high socioeconomic deprivation. *Journal of Comorbidity* 2017;7:1–10.

18. http://www.healthscotland.scot/publications/evaluation-of-the-links-worker-programme-in-deep-end-general-practices-in-glasgow

3.5 Caring

1. Mercer SM, Watt GCM. The Inverse Care Law: Clinical primary care encounters in deprived and affluent areas of Scotland. *Annals of Family Medicine* 2007;5:503–510.

2. Pioneers. The Good Doctor, BBC2, 7 Oct 1996.

3. Tudor Hart J, Dieppe P. Caring effects. *Lancet* 1996;347:1606–1608.

4. Collings JS. General practice in England today: A reconnaissance. *Lancet* 1950;i:555–585.

5. NHS National Services Scotland. Practice team information (PTI). Annual update (2012/13). Information Services Division, 29 October 2013. http://www.isdscotland.org/Health-Topics/General-Practice/Publications/2013-10-29/2013-10-29-PTI-Report.pdf.

6. Watt G. The Inverse Care Law today. *Lancet* 2002;360:252–254.

3.6 Continuity

1. Hart JT. *A New Kind of Doctor: The General Practitioner's Part in the Health of the Community.* Merlin Press, London, UK, 1988. p. 187.

2. Hart JT, Thomas C, Gibbons B, Edwards C, Hart M, Jones J, Jones M, Walton P. Twenty five years of case-finding and audit in a socially-deprived community. *BMJ* 1991;302:1509–1513.

3. Pereira Gray DJ, Sidaway-Lee K, White E, Thorne A, Evans PH. Continuity of care with doctors—a matter of life and death? A systematic review of continuity of care and mortality. *BMJ Open* 2018;e021161. doi:10.1136/bmjopen-2017-021161.

3.7 Coordination

1. Cairns D. *The Memoirs of Hector Berlioz*. Sphere Books, London, UK, 1990.

3.8 Coverage

1. Hart JT. Measurement of omission. *British Medical Journal* 1982;284:1686–1689.

3.9 Clinical generalism in Scotland

1. Gillies J, Mercer S, Lyon A, Scott M, Watt G. Distilling the essence of general practice. *BJGP* 2009;59:e167–e176.
2. Reeve J. Protecting generalism: Moving on from evidence-based medicine. *BJGP* 2010;60:521–523.
3. De Maeseneer J. Multimorbidity, goal-oriented care and equity. The RCGP James MacKenzie lecture. *BJGP* 2012;62:e522–e524.
4. Gillies J. (Ed.). *RCGP Scotland: The First 60 Years*. Royal College of General Practitioners (Scotland), Edinburgh, UK, 2013.
5. Howie J, Whitfield M. *Academic General Practice in the UK Medical Schools, 1948–2000: A Short History*. Edinburgh University Press, Edinburgh, UK, 2011.
6. GPs at the Deep End. https://www.gla.ac.uk/researchinstitutes/healthwellbeing/research/generalpracticedeepend/.
7. The Highlands and Islands Medical Service. http://www.ournhsscotland.com/history/birth-nhs-scotland/highlands-and-islands-medical-service (Accessed 4th September 2018.)
8. "Dewar 2012". http://ruralgp.com/dewar2012/ (Accessed 4th September 2018.)
9. Barnett K, Mercer SW, Norbury M, Watt G, Wyke S, Guthrie B. Epidemiology of multimorbidity and implications for health care, research, and medical education: A cross-sectional study. *Lancet* 2012;380:37–43.
10. Hart JT. The Inverse Care Law. *Lancet* 1971;297:405–412.
11. Chief Medical Officer's Annual Report 2014–2015. *Realistic Medicine*. Scottish Government, Edinburgh, UK, 2016.
12. Chief Medical Officer's Annual Report 2015–2016. *Realising Realistic Medicine*. Scottish Government, Edinburgh, UK, 2017.
13. Guthrie B, Gillies J, Calderwood C, Smith G, Mercer S. Developing middle ground research to support primary care transformation. *BJGP* 2017;67:498–499.
14. BMA Scotland/Scottish Government. *The 2018 General Medical Services Contract in Scotland*. Scottish Government, Edinburgh, UK, 2017.

4

Pioneers

The history of general practice is full of pioneers, mostly unrecorded and unsung, who made a difference where they worked for the best of motives and with no thought of recognition or reward.

A few pioneers are identifiable, however, because of what they wrote or was written about them and the influence their examples have had either directly on practice or in showing what it is possible for general practitioners to do.

The following pioneering examples concern research, the population approach and advocacy.

4.1 PIONEERS IN RESEARCH

Research usually begins with an idea about what is happening, why it is happening or how things could be improved ('seeing what others have seen, thinking what nobody has thought'), followed by a structured enquiry to establish whether the initial conjecture is true. A clear answer does not guarantee a clear question. However, if the study has been well designed and carried out, the researcher can report the findings to the outside world, usually in a scientific journal after passing the peer review process.

4.1.1 Edward Jenner (1749–1823)

One of the first GP researchers was Edward Jenner, a country doctor who practiced in Berkeley, Gloucestershire and was a member of the Gloucestershire Medical Society which met at the Fleece Inn in Rodborough to present and discuss their conjectures and findings. On 14 May 1796, he inoculated an eight-year-old boy James Phipps with scraped pus from cowpox blisters on the hands of Sarah Nelmes, a milkmaid who had caught cowpox from a cow called Blossom. Jenner was not the first person to inoculate patients with cowpox (as a child he had been inoculated himself). However, by proving with subsequent challenges that inoculated patients were then immune to smallpox, he was largely responsible for this finding being accepted and applied (although not immediately – he was ridiculed at first). It was not Jenner's first foray into medical research. He had previously postulated that angina pectoris was a consequence of coronary atheroma. In 1792, he obtained his MD from the University of St Andrews. Probably, no subsequent GP researcher has saved as many lives as Edward Jenner.

4.1.2 Sir James Mackenzie (1853–1925)

Born in Scone, Perthshire and a graduate of the University of Edinburgh, James Mackenzie practiced for many years as a GP in Burnley, Lancashire where many of his patients worked in the cotton mills and lived in very poor housing conditions (1). It is remarkable that he carried out research in such a setting, and the nature of his studies was astonishing – for example, observing and analysing the behaviour of the jugular venous pulse in patients with heart disease. By noticing the absence of *a* waves in patients with an irregularly irregular pulse, he was the first person to observe and explain atrial fibrillation. He corresponded with the leading cardiologists and electrophysiologists of his day in the United Kingdom and abroad. On moving to London, he became more of a cardiologist than a general practitioner and was knighted for his work.

Mackenzie always had the idea that general practice was the ideal setting in which to observe and address the early origins of disease and when he retired to St Andrews in Fife it was to set up an Institute to carry out such research in partnership with local general practitioners. The initiative did not prosper following Mackenzie's death, but it did inspire a visiting US cardiologist Paul White who 20 years later was one of the originators of the Framingham Study in Massachusetts, one of the longest and most productive cohort studies, especially concerning cardiovascular risks.

A paper in the *British Medical Journal* on 4 June 1921, defending the thesis 'that the opportunities of the general practitioner are essential for the investigation of disease and the progress of medicine' gives a clear picture of Sir James Mackenzie and his thinking. Addressing a mostly specialist audience, he concluded,

> I know quite well that these views at present will fail to carry conviction. All I wish you to do is to pause from time to time and ask whether they are true. (2)

4.1.3 William Pickles (1885–1969)

William Pickles was a general practitioner at Aysgarth in the Yorkshire Dales for over 50 years beginning in 1912.

Pickles demonstrated that by collecting simple information from a practice over many years, it is possible to make important discoveries concerning the nature of health and illness in local communities. This work was helped by his long-term knowledge of patients and families, and by the natural bonds of goodwill and helpfulness that exist between local communities and their general practitioners.

In a self-contained community, where travel was limited and incomers were few, Pickles used local knowledge to track and explain the incidence and spread of infection, providing original information on the incubation periods of several infectious diseases, such as Bornholm's disease and hepatitis. He was 45 years old when his first paper from practice was published.

His biographer John Pemberton records how Pickles developed a simple but useful method of charting all the new cases of infectious disease that he saw (3). Each new case was noted down in his pocket diary with the name, place and date of onset. The information was transferred by his wife to a time chart on which the villages that made up the practice were kept separate. About once a fortnight, the charts were brought up to date. Each disease had its own coloured symbol. Over the first 20 years of his observations, 6808 cases of the infectious disease were recorded. From these charts and his intimate knowledge of the lives of his patients, Pickles was often able to trace the source and spread of epidemics in the Dale, always on the lookout for what he called 'the short and only possible contact.'

What he did was extraordinary, but he did it in an ordinary place and his methods were simple. Several other GPs, including John Fry (4) and Keith Hodgkin (5), followed his example by collecting practice data over a long period of time to obtain otherwise unknowable perspectives about the nature of health and illness in practice populations. Franz Huygen, a Dutch GP, used a similar approach in charting the occurrence of illnesses in successive generations of families (6).

Pickles is not known for family studies. However, in 1943, he published a paper in the *Lancet* (7), which mapped the occurrence of rheumatic heart disease in 23 out of 53 descendants of an incident case. He wrote:

> After 30 years' close experience, I have no hesitation in singling these people out as among the most outstanding in the district. With insignificant exceptions they are prosperous, well-housed and well-fed. They are as a rule, successful farmers, but a switch over to other occupations has simply meant adaptation of talents and successes in a new sphere. Yet none of these sufferers has up to the present died from heart disease at an early age. It may be that the environment has hitherto been so favourable for this family that it has helped family members in part to elude the shackles of inheritance.

Families share environments and habits, as well as their genes, and it is the interaction that counts. Pickles' observation and insight remind us that there is more to life, health and illness than the genetic prescription with which we are born(8).

4.1.4 Seizing opportunities

The examples of Jenner, Mackenzie and Pickles reflect the times when they lived and the circumstances in which they worked. Nowadays, it is very unusual for single researchers to make discoveries on their own, but it is not impossible.

Following Pickles' example, Robert Hope Simpson recorded 192 cases of herpes zoster (shingles) in his Cirencester general practice between 1947 and 1962 (9).

He found that the severity increased with age. However, the condition did not occur in epidemics, and there was no characteristic seasonal variation. A low prevalence of varicella (chickenpox) was associated with a high incidence of zoster. He is credited with showing that shingles is caused by a reactivation of the chicken pox virus.

Julian Tudor Hart and Mary Thomas met as members of Archie Cochrane's team at the MRC Epidemiology Unit in South Wales which in the 1950s galvanised whole communities for medical research, regularly achieves response rates of over 90% (10). But Julian was frustrated by research rules, which meant that while he often observed gross pathology in participants, he could not intervene. So, he left to set up practice at Glyncorrwg, a mining village in West Glamorgan, exchanging 'a life of facts for the facts of life', applying not only the epidemiological approach to clinical practice but also Cochrane's magic ingredient, the employment of local people who were streetwise and knew their communities well.

In a series of practice-based studies with very high response rates, Glyncorrwg became the pilot site for many of the early studies of the MRC general practice research framework, including a survey of urinary incontinence, collection of stool samples for a prospective study of faecal flora and bowel cancer and community dietary salt restriction to intakes below 3 g per day (11). The doctor went the extra mile in delivering health care; patients went the extra mile in taking part in research. While the Welsh coal industry went into decline, Tudor Hart was mining a hugely productive alternative energy source.

Responding to an imminent factory closure which would put many of his patients out of work, Norman Beale at Calne in Wiltshire set up a cohort study in which he monitored his patients' use of services before and after the closure (12). He showed that the main psychological and other effects on patients' health occurred in anticipation of the closure rather than when the closure had occurred.

Roy Robertson at the Muirhouse practice in Edinburgh, serving a very deprived housing estate, had a large number of patients who were injecting drug misusers (13). As part of their care, he had collected a bank of stored serum samples. When the HIV epidemic arrived, this cohort and bank of baseline samples became a unique resource for studying the natural history of HIV in drug misusers. Even after 30 years, the cohort continues. Roy Robertson was made a Fellow of the Royal Society of Edinburgh.

Jim Douglas at Fort William in the Highlands of Scotland (Section 3.10) noticed a higher prevalence of asthma in his patients who worked at a local fish processing factory. By investigating their health and environmental exposure at work and linking with immunologists at the University of Glasgow, he demonstrated not only their allergy to antigens in processed salmon but also a marked reduction in asthma prevalence when aerosols transmitting the allergen were controlled. Like Cronin's GP hero in *The Citadel*, Jim Douglas obtained an MD degree for his practice-based research but, going one better, his results were published in the *Lancet* (14).

4.1.5 University-based research

Most higher research degrees (i.e. MD or PhD) obtained by general practitioners are now based on some kind of university attachment at the outset of their careers. Between 1974 and 2016 in Scotland, the number of higher research degrees obtained by general practitioners working from their practice without a university appointment could be counted on the fingers of one hand.

Participation in research has increased, however, largely due to the development of networks of research practices which have made it possible to recruit patients and apply a wide variety of research protocols for epidemiological, health services and clinical research. Practices are usually involved in delivery rather than research design.

An exception was the Care Plus Study (15) involving a randomised controlled trial of extended consultations for complex patients in general practices serving very deprived areas in Glasgow (Section 3.4). In contrast to most research studies, funding was obtained before it was possible to agree either the case definition or the nature of the intervention. Both had to be developed in consultation with the participating practices after they had been recruited. Whether this process of emergent co-design is considered a valuable precedent remains to be seen.

4.2 POPULATION MEDICINE

Universal registration of patients in general practices in the UK National Health Service provides not only population contact and cumulative coverage but also continuity and high levels of public trust. These are huge resources that can be harnessed for the public good. No other public service has these attributes. The pioneer of population medicine in the United Kingdom was Dr Julian Tudor Hart.

4.2.1 Career advice for medical students

I work in a colliery practice – an industrial village with only one doctor and 2,000 patients. Not one is a stranger; they are not only patients but fellow citizens. From many direct and indirect contacts, many non-medical though shared activities, schools, shops, and gossip, I have come to understand how ignorant I would be if I knew them only as a doctor seeing them when they were ill. It is a compact world, in which integrity and a sense of proportion are more easily retained than in cities, provided that one accepts the multiple faces one must wear in an intimate communal life. There is immense friendliness, much bravery and generosity, a good deal of petty meanness, treachery, and servile cowardice – but never indifference.

This is in many ways the ideal setting for primary care, particularly when combined with research. It is the only situation in which the skills of epidemiology and clinical medicine can be practiced by one person, in which observation, experiment and action can be combined and in which major discoveries are still possible by a few people with simple equipment. This is so also in truly rural practice, but despite the idyllic life this can afford, numbers are bound to be smaller and more scattered, and the generally good standard of health in the country may be a smaller challenge than the higher illness rates and mortality of industrial areas. Colliery practices are semi-rural isolates of the situation in the industrial areas of cities, with deep-rooted traditions of insufficient medical care, overworked doctors, and a low level of health education, a great deal of serious illness and serious social problems. These conditions make the greatest demands but can also yield the greatest satisfactions to young doctors committed to primary care. There are very real difficulties of isolation from professional colleagues (much less now than it was) and hospital support is less comprehensive and less accessible than students learn to expect in teaching hospitals.

With great effort, any doctor can get to know all his patients, even in a city with high migrant turnover. Only thus can he learn to think in terms of a responsibility not only to the patient sitting in the surgery but to the whole population for whose care he is paid and for whose health he is responsible. He can then see his role as the ultimate custodian of the public health on a defined section of a world front against misery and disease. All of this is a great deal easier when this population is visibly and tangibly defined, whether as a dispersed rural community, a compact industrial village, a part of a large council housing estate or one of those traditional neighbourhoods that still persist in some central areas of cities. To know every patient and many of his relatives, friends and workmates mean that you see him as an individual with a medical and social history which hints at a particular set of risks for the future. You have the information and the motivation to try to prevent disease by a continual quiet search for underlying causes and for reversible stages in possibly lethal or disabling sequences of causation. To me this is the most exciting and satisfying part of medicine, and probably one of its major growing points during the next 30 years.

The greatest rewards in primary care are going to be found in those areas that most need good doctoring, but which at present are least likely to get it. To do this one must discard the sorts of ambition still encouraged by some teaching hospitals. We need more liberty, more equality but above all more fraternity; the doctor living and working within a community, sharing as much as he can of the common experience, is better able than any other to discard privilege and stand on two firm legs of earned respect.

Julian Tudor Hart
Lancet Career Guide for Medical Students, 1973 (1)
Reproduced with permission of *The Lancet*

4.2.2 The example of Julian Tudor Hart

Fahrenheit 451, the title of a book by Ray Bradbury and film by François Truffaut, records the temperature at which paper burns. In a totalitarian state where books were burned, each member of the resistance was tasked with remembering one book, to keep its story alive. As the future of primary care depends so much on health practitioners, and how they see their work, the Glyncorrwg story is the one they need to know, not only how it started but also how it may carry on.

So much of what Julian Tudor Hart pioneered at Glyncorrwg, a former mining village in South Wales, is orthodox now. He was the first doctor to measure the blood pressures of all his patients (2). Famously, the last man to take part, who only agreed to take part if he was the only person who hadn't, had the highest blood pressure of all, which remains an important teaching lesson. Julian and his wife, Mary, put their records into shape, converting from Lloyd George to A4, and then to computerised records, to establish the information system that allowed them to start by screening the records, not the patients; and to measure what they had not done (the 'measurement of omission') (3), so they could describe, address and reduce the 'rule of halves' (4). Later, Julian could describe a cohort of patients with hypertension diagnosed at <40 years of age and follow up over 20 years (5); be 'his own coroner', reviewing over 500 consecutive deaths in general practice (6); and assess his impact on premature mortality after 25 years of practice (7).

All this had an impact via research articles, opinion pieces and books, but also by example. The 1991 *BMJ* paper is still the only paper in the literature which reports what a GP might achieve in a lifetime's practice (7). Even with wide confidence limits, the observed 30% lower premature mortality was quite an effect, achieved not only via the delivery of evidence-based medicine (before statins) as promulgated today by NICE and enshrined in the QOF – but also, importantly, and outside the QOF, via unconditional, personalised continuity of care provided for all patients regardless of whatever problem or combination of problems they presented. Achieving this in one of the most deprived areas in West Glamorgan demonstrated that the Inverse Care Law (Section 5.7) is not a law of nature (8), but a state of affairs that can be reversed.

4.3 ADVOCACY

The social causes of illness are just as important as the physical ones. Aetiological therapy means more than killing a few bugs. The medical officer of health and the practitioners of a distressed area are the natural advocates of the people. They well know the factors that paralyse all their efforts. They are not only scientists but also responsible citizens and if they did not raise their voice, who else should?

H. E. Sigerist (1)

* The text of Section 4.2.2 is taken from an article published in the *British Journal of General Practice*. Watt G. 8th Julian Tudor Hart Lecture 2014: Include me out, exclude you in. *Br J Gen Pract* 2015. doi:10.3399/bjgp15X686317.

The simplest and most elemental aspect of advocacy in general practice lies in being ambitious for the patients' health, imagining what can be achieved and how, going the extra mile and ensuring that what could and should happen does happen.

Of course, many factors influencing health operate outside health care. As Sigerist wrote, general practitioners well know the factors that paralyse all their efforts. The question is 'What can they do?'

4.3.1 Dr Lachlan Grant (1871–1945)

JAMES D. M. DOUGLAS

Dr Lachlan Grant (Figure 4.1) practiced as a general practitioner in the remote community of Ballachulish in the Scottish Highlands for 40 years. He set out his ideas for a National Health Service in 1912, 36 years before its foundation.

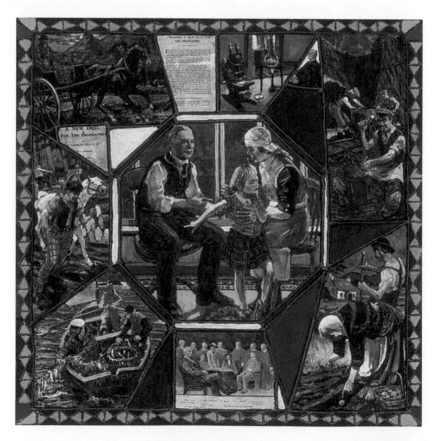

Figure 4.1 This painting of Dr Lachlan Grant by Alastair Smyth was commissioned by Dr James Douglas as a gift to display in RCGP Scotland on the centenary of the "Dewar Report" in 2012.

Lachlan Grant was raised and schooled in Ballachulish. He spoke Gaelic and loved Scottish culture. He became a prize-winning medical student and could have followed a medical career with status in the city. Instead, he prepared himself with a broad range of hospital jobs and returned to his home village. He expressed a clear mission to serve 'his community'.

After school, he had worked in the slate quarry to finance his university studies and returned as the 'company doctor'. He was employed by the quarry and expected to provide medical care to the workers and their families. The booming industry was providing roofing slate for industrial Glasgow.

He twice challenged the company on workers' safety issues and was sacked on both occasions. The employees came out on strike to support him and twice he was reinstated.

He had been established in practice for seven years when the government 'Dewar Commission' Section 3.9 took evidence throughout the Highlands and Islands on the difficulties of providing a health service to remote communities. His evidence was recorded along with many other doctors and community leaders.

His evidence stands out because he moved quickly from re-stating problems to offering solutions. The people had no money to pay the doctors' fees. Rural poverty, endemic disease and poor-quality doctors were the challenges.

He set out a clear vision for a 'National Health Service' in 1912 with doctor's tenure subsidised by the government. He articulated the 'essentiality' of medical provision in communities where the people had no means to pay. A hundred years ago, he described the public health systems, patient education, professional education and governance that we have today.

He was interested in medical science. He established his own laboratory for the diagnosis of TB. Aluminium smelting came as a source of new employment but had to be considered as a potential occupational poison. He published the evidence of safety from his practice population.

Grant was a polymath and community leader. His political campaigns included rural poverty, rural depopulation, unemployment, industrial investment and workers collectivism. The foundation of these inspiring ideas came from his clinical general practice and his desire to improve the health of his remote community.

4.3.2 Direct action for public health

In King Vidor's film of *The Citadel,* based on the novel by A. J. Cronin, starring Robert Donat and Rosalind Russell, two GPs float dynamite in cocoa tins down a sewer, blowing it up so that it had to be replaced (2). The leaking sewer was contaminating the local water supply and causing cases of paratyphoid in their patients, but the doctors had no success in getting officialdom to replace the sewer. Hence they resorted to desperate measures.

As with so many of Cronin's medical stories, it had a basis in fact. After months of searching through local papers at the British Library's newsroom, the *Lancet's* Ruth Richardson found the following news report in the *South Wales Argus* of 29 September 1923 (3).

> ### BOX 4.1: Road blown up
>
> *Alarming gas explosion at Bedwas*
>
> Some consternation was caused early on Sunday morning at Bedwas by an explosion which blew up a considerable portion of Church Street, the main thoroughfare. It was caused by an escape of gas from the main into a culvert. The culvert was ripped open for a distance of between 60 and 100 yards. Fortunately, no one was injured.

Richardson commented,

> There are probably people in Bedwas who recollect that local miners detonated the sewer at the behest of 'Doc' Bob Roberts, well known as a doughty fighter for his patient's health. Cronin's admiration for Roberts's breed of preventive medicine is inscribed in the novel.

If there have been other examples of GPs taking direct action in this way, they go unrecorded.

4.3.3 Advocating for a National Health Service

Will Pickles argued for a National Health Service and was not afraid of the unpopularity this brought him from within the profession. He detested the financial aspects of general practice which involved, in addition to borrowing money to buy a practice, the business of trying to collect bad debts, sometimes by employing debt collectors. As with many other doctors, a financial relationship between doctor and patient seemed to interfere with the doctor–patient relationship. In a lecture to the Socialist Medical Association, Pickles said of past conditions (4),

> The monetary aspect of the practice had to be of supreme importance and I can see that it might have become the ruling passion of one's life. There certainly was at the end of those twenty years a feeling of satisfaction in one's emancipation and I am bound to say a feeling of pride in at last owning the freehold of one's practice. But looking back I do not think that the heavy burden of debt was conducive to a detached attitude to one's work and the making of money simply had to be rather prominent.
>
> For many years, ever since the dawn of proposals for a National Health Service my colleagues, all country practitioners in virtually unopposed practices, have met in my house and in a most friendly and unofficial way discussed the various aspects of the subject. The attendances would average twelve and although rather more than half would fall in the upper age group the younger men were

well represented. At the outset we felt that we were not now able to do all that we would wish for our patients in the way of specialists and hospital services and that, we were ashamed to have to acknowledge it, we could do a great deal more for those whose pockets were reasonably well lined than for those whose pockets were not. The hopelessly long wait that there is before one could get a young man operated on for a hernia or a child for the removal of tonsils and adenoids would be instances.

We had hopes that a National Health Service would fulfil these wants and we felt that the present time gave the profession a glorious opportunity for putting its house in order.

Pickles was also in favour of a full-time salaried service:

The fairest arrangement is a full-time salaried service. I say this after years of thought and not always with this decision. I used to think it would encourage the slacker, but I have come to the conclusion that the real slacker is the man who takes 4,000 on his list and does the minimum for them. (4)

These views were not popular at that time. The issue of salaried service remains controversial. When the College of General Practitioners was founded in 1952, twenty years before 'Royal' could be added, Pickles was its first President.

The next examples of advocacy come from the Deep End Project (see Section 6.1) involving general practices serving the 100 most deprived communities in Scotland.

4.3.4 Welfare reform

In 2012, General Practitioners at the Deep End produced a report on their experiences of the impact of austerity on patients and general practices in very deprived areas (4).

Concerns had been raised about the consequences of the government's welfare reforms and other austerity measures. These concerns included the negative impact that cuts in benefits were having on some of the society's most vulnerable individuals and families.

GPs were asked to reflect on the effects of austerity measures on patients and on patient care in the previous week.

Most of the issues raised were related to the direct and indirect effects of austerity policies including benefit cuts, service cutbacks and an increasing number of patients being taken off Employment Support Allowance (ESA) or Disability Living Allowance (DLA). The issues can be divided into those affecting patients, practices, secondary care/support services and social work/ housing.

A central concern of Deep End practitioners was the number of patients with deteriorating mental health. At one end of the spectrum, there were those in work, previously well but under increasing stress and job insecurity due to cutbacks and taking on extra work/jobs, with resultant impacts on family and relationships.

At the other end of the spectrum, there were those deemed 'fit for work', who had their benefits cut and then struggled to make ends meet, resulting in increasing contact with GPs and psychiatrists, increasing use of antidepressant and antipsychotic drugs and increasing self-medication with drugs and alcohol.

Aside from the direct detrimental effects of drugs, alcohol and worsening mental health on physical health, patients' health could be affected indirectly as many patients were reluctant to take time off work due to job insecurity. Additionally, GPs reported less time in consultations to deal with physical problems, as these were no longer a priority for the patient.

> I observe this again and again that I cannot address medical issues as I have to deal with the patient's agenda first, which is getting money to feed and heat.

Financial hardship was manifested in several ways, but perhaps the most striking was the growing number of individuals and families experiencing fuel poverty – the combination of increased costs and falling benefits resulting in a choice between heating and eating. Practices reported cases of an elderly patient going to a friend's house in order to wash; families relying on relatives to pay for food and cigarettes (unable to stop smoking due to stress) and a mother resorting to prostitution to feed herself and her family.

> In my surgery, I am hearing from patients who for two to three days a week cannot afford to heat their houses (many use metered cards which are more expensive than direct debit payments).

Changes to the benefits system were cited by most GP respondents as impacting on patients' health and practice workload. Practices described an 'endless cycle' of appeals, during which patients' benefit payments were reduced.

> For obvious reasons the patients in X (deprived area of Glasgow) call Corunna House (where the Work Capability Assessments are done) 'Lourdes' because all the sick come out cured!

Most patients appealed WCA decisions and asked their GPs for letters in support. This was encouraged by benefit support workers and solicitors with impacts on practice time that would otherwise have been spent on health issues.

Practices reported frustration among staff at their inability to alleviate the suffering they saw and increased stress due to extra workload.

Patient transport for outpatient appointments had been affected by cutbacks, such that there were reports of patients complaining about long waits, with some elderly frail patients arriving home after midnight.

Addiction workers were said to be struggling to do any structured addiction work with patients because they were too busy trying to help patients in crisis.

Patients attended Community Addiction Teams for crisis loans due to their benefits being cut, but addiction and social services had run out of funds.

One respondent felt that GP practices were a 'dumping ground', as other services were affected by cutbacks and withdrew from care.

Social work was described as a service that is overworked, understaffed and ultimately failing some of the most vulnerable members of society. There were reports of vulnerable adults and children being unallocated despite serious concerns for their safety and/or well-being, difficulty getting social work colleagues to attend practice meetings, increased difficulty getting patients into respite care and increasing reliance on the voluntary sector.

Addiction services and social services had been told to turn to charities for basic items such as beds and cookers when children were returned from care to their parents.

> We have a working single mother who became homeless due to community violence. She has been in a cold damp flat sleeping on a mattress on the floor with her 11-month-old child for nearly six months. Housing has been unable to find her a suitable flat.

The report travelled like wildfire, quickly arriving on Minister's desks at Holyrood and Westminster. Its novelty, topicality and authority resulted in invitations to meet politicians and civil servants, several of whom admitted that they had underestimated the mental health effects of welfare reforms.

Deep End Reports 21, 25 and 27 continued this theme (5–7), resulting finally in the Deep End Advice Worker Project (Section 14.2).

4.3.5 Alcohol in general practice

The following letter, signed by 41 general practitioners, was published in the *Herald* newspaper in the week that a proposal for minimum alcohol pricing was being debated in the Scottish Parliament (8).

> We write as general practitioners working in the most deprived areas of Scotland, with special experience of the problems of alcohol. Our interest is not through choice, but because of the huge, recent and increasing importance of excessive alcohol consumption as a cause of premature death, physical illness and social harm affecting our young patients.
>
> Research studies show the social patterning of alcohol problems, not only the higher levels of consumption in poor areas but also the higher levels of harm for a given level of consumption. Death rates from alcohol liver disease are five times more common in poor areas compared with the most affluent areas.
>
> Scotland's statistics are shocking, but 'statistics are people with the tears wiped off'. The current debate about alcohol pricing can lose sight of the misery and devastation that affects our

patients and their families, especially the lasting effects on children. Drunken disorder is only the most obvious problem. Every one of us knows of tragic cases of young adults whose lives, and whose family lives, have been ruined by alcohol. Women are particularly vulnerable. No one should die young and yellow from chronic alcohol poisoning.

This is not an issue that can be left to personal responsibility or the massed efforts of health practitioners trying to stem the tide. Any measure, such as minimal alcohol pricing, which makes it more difficult for people to consume regular excessive amounts of alcohol should be seized as a public health measure of the highest importance. Cross-party support is the least we should expect from our politicians, especially those representing the most deprived constituencies, in confronting this very real and lethal epidemic.

After a long process of unsuccessful legal appeals by the alcohol industry, including an application to the Supreme Court, the Scottish Government introduced minimum unit pricing for alcohol on 1 May 2018.

> It is the greatest of all mistakes to do nothing because you can only do a little. Do what you can.
>
> **Sydney Smith**

REFERENCES

4.1 Pioneers in research

1. Mair A. *James Mackenzie MD General Practitioner 1853–1925*. Churchill Livingstone, London, UK, 1973.
2. Mackenzie J. A defence of the thesis that 'the opportunities of the general practitioner are essential for the investigation of disease and the progress of medicine'. *Br Med J* 1921;1:797–804. https://www.ncbi.nlm.nih.gov/pmc/articles/PMC2415240/pdf/brmedj06694-0003.pdf
3. Pemberton J. *Will Pickles of Wensleydale. The Life of a Country Doctor*. Royal College of General Practitioners, London, UK, 1984.
4. Fry J. *Common Diseases: Their Nature, Incidence and Care*. Lippincott, Philadelphia, PA, 1979.
5. Hodgkin K. *Towards Earlier Diagnosis in Primary Care*. Churchill Livingstone, Edinburgh, UK, 1978.
6. Huygen FJA. *Family Medicine. The Medical Life History of Families*. Royal College of General Practitioners, London, UK, 1990.

7. Pickles WN. A rheumatic family. *Lancet* 1943;2:241.
8. Watt G. General practice and the epidemiology of health and disease in families. RCGP Pickles Lecture 2004. *Br J Gen Pract* 2004;54:939–944.
9. Hope Simpson RE. The nature of herpes zoster: A long-term study and a new hypothesis. *Proc Roy Soc Med* 1965;58:9–20.
10. Hart JT, Davey Smith G. Response rates in South Wales 1950–1996: Changing requirements for mass participation in human research. In: Chalmers I, Maynard A (Eds.), *Non-random Reflections on Health Services Research: On the 25th Anniversary of Archie Cochrane's Effectiveness & Efficiency.* BMJ Publishing Group, London, UK, 1997. pp. 31–57.
11. Watt GCM, Foy CJW, Hart JT Bingham G, Edwards C, Hart M, Thomas E, Walton P. Dietary sodium and arterial blood pressure: Evidence against genetic susceptibility. *Br Med J (Clin Res Ed)* 1985;291:1525–1528.
12. Beale N, Nethercott S. Job-loss and morbidity in a group of employees nearing retirement age. *J Roy Coll Gen Pract* 1986;36:265–266.
13. Kimber J, Copeland L, Hickman M, Macleod J, McKenzie J, De Angelis D, Robertson JR. Survival and cessation in injecting drug users: Prospective observational study of outcomes and effect of opiate substitution treatment. *BMJ* 2011;351. doi:10.1136/bmj.c3712.
14. Douglas JDM, McSharry C, Blaikie L, Morrow T, Miles S, Franklin D. Occupational asthma caused by automated salmon processing. *Lancet* 1995;346:737–740.
15. Mercer SW, Fitzpatrick B, Guthrie B, Fenwick E, Grieve E, Lawson K, Boyer N et al. The CARE Plus study – A whole system intervention to improve quality of life of primary care patients with multimorbidity in areas of high socioeconomic deprivation: Cluster randomised controlled trial. *BMC Med* 2016;14:88.

4.2 Population medicine

1. Hart JT. *Lancet Career Guide for Medical Students.* Lancet Publications, London, UK, 1973.
2. Hart JT. Semi-continuous screening of a whole community for hypertension. *Lancet* 1970;2:223–226.
3. Hart JT. Measurement of omission. *Br Med J (Clin Res Ed)* 1982;284:1686–1689.
4. Hart JT. Rule of halves: Implications of under-diagnosis and dropout for future workload and prescribing costs in primary care. *Br J Gen Pract* 1992;42:116–119.
5. Hart JT, Edwards C, Hart M, Jones J, Jones M, Haines AP, Watt G. Screen detected high blood pressure under 40: A general practice population followed up for 21 years. *BMJ* 1993;306:437–444.
6. Hart JT, Humphreys C. Be your own coroner: An audit of 500 consecutive deaths in a general practice. *Br Med J (Clin Res Ed)* 1987;294:871–874.

7. Hart JT, Thomas C, Gibbons B, Edwards C, Hart M, Jones J, Jones M, Walton P. Twenty-five years of case-finding and audit in a socially-deprived community. *BMJ* 1991;302:1509–1513.
8. Hart JT. The Inverse Care Law. *Lancet* 1971;1:405–412.

4.3 Advocacy

1. Sigerist HE. *Medicine and Human Welfare*. Yale University Press, New Haven, CT, 1941.
2. Richardson R. AJ Cronin's The Citadel. *Lancet* 2016;387:2284–2285.
3. Pemberton, J. *Will Pickles of Wensleydale. The Life of a Country Doctor*. Royal College of General Practitioners, London, UK, 1984.
4. Deep End Report 16. GPs at the Deep End Austerity Report. March 2012. www.gla.ac.uk/deepend.
5. Deep End Report 21. GP experience of welfare reform in very deprived areas. October 2013. www.gla.ac.uk/deepend.
6. Deep End Report 25. Strengthening primary care partnership responses to the welfare reforms. November 2014. www.gla.ac.uk/deepend.
7. Deep End Report 27. Improving partnership working between general practices and financial advice services in Glasgow: One year on. December 2015. www.gla.ac.uk/deepend.
8. General Practitioners at the Deep End. Alcohol in general practice (letter). *The Herald*, 13 September 2010.

5

Challenges

This section covers some of the important challenges facing health systems. After a brief review of confusing terminology, Stewart Mercer describes the epidemiology of multimorbidity. Following a section that considers the challenge of multimorbidity for health services, Ken Mclean considers how to assess the quality of generalist clinical care. The next sections consider reasons for the imbalance between specialist and generalist care, how sufficient numbers of generalists can be maintained and the continuing challenge of health inequalities as a result of the Inverse Care Law. Finally, Breannon Babbel reports the views of general practitioners as to whether and how they can address inequalities in health.

5.1 CONFUSING TERMINOLOGY

When I use a word,' Humpty Dumpty said, in rather a scornful tone, 'it means just what I choose it to mean—neither more nor less.
The question is,' said Alice, 'whether you can make words mean so many different things.'
'The question is,' said Humpty Dumpty, 'which is to be master—that's all.

Lewis Carroll
Through the Looking Glass

Terminology is confusing when the same term is used to describe different things and thus has a different meaning for different people.

Primary care is such a term, referring variously to a place, to types of professionals and to function. Referring to place, primary care is often used to refer to everything that happens in health care outside the hospital. Referring to people, primary care refers to health professionals who work outside hospitals. Referring to function, primary care as defined by Barbara Starfield is characterised by first contact, continuity, comprehensiveness and coordination. This functional definition is much narrower than the WHO definition of primary care as promulgated in its 1978 Alma-Ata Declaration, in which primary care was more or less synonymous with public health, including education, the environment and economy in addition to health care services.

Universal health coverage is a similarly vague term, not specifying what conditions and treatments are covered for which people. Most countries provide universal coverage for road accidents and other emergencies but can differ hugely in terms of access to continuing care and specialist investigations and treatment. Universal coverage can provide access to care, but not needs-based care when resources are insufficient to provide the investigations and treatments that patients need.

The **Inverse Care Law** states that the availability of good medical care tends to vary inversely with the need for it in the population served. However, the term is often used loosely as a synonym for inequalities in health or accepted as a law of nature rather than a man-made set of arrangements which restricts needs-based care. General Practitioners at the Deep End (see Section 6.1) contend that the Inverse Care Law is not about good medical care in some areas and bad medical care in other; rather, it is about the difference between what they can do and what they could do for patients with additional resources.

Concepts such as **Quality Health care** and **Realistic Medicine** seldom take into account what constitutes quality and realism in different contexts; for example, in parts of the service which are time-poor, where the burden of multimorbidity and social complexity is high or where patients have less health literacy, confidence and agency.

Anticipatory care, as introduced by the Dutch general practitioner Van Der Dool (1), originally referred to the use of routine encounters in general practice to address preventive issues in addition to the issues presented on the day by patients. More recently, anticipatory care refers to the eliciting of patients' preferences regarding end-of-life care.

Personalised medicine, which many consider the hallmark of generalist clinical practice, is now often bowdlerised as a synonym for 'precision medicine' whereby patients are included or excluded from treatment according to their genotype.

Patient-centred medicine is professed by all health professionals and services, but patients are not always at the centre, especially when care is fragmented with multimorbid patients receiving care from many different clinics.

Specialist colleagues working with general practice teams are variously described as **'co-located'**, **'attached'** or **'embedded'** with different meanings and implications for working relationships and accountability.

An army of new professional staff has been created recently with job titles including **'link workers'**, **'community link practitioners'**, **'community organisers'**, **'navigators'** and **'networkers'**, with job descriptions comprising various combinations of 'social prescribing' and patient support (Section 8.2).

The response to ambiguous and confusing terminologies has to be 'what do you mean' and 'what do you actually do?'

5.2 MULTIMORBIDITY

STEWART W. MERCER

The epidemiology of multimorbidity was investigated in Scotland using routine primary care electronic data and published in the *Lancet* in 2012 (1). Since then the paper has been cited over 2,000 times and has had a major influence on policy in the United Kingdom and internationally. The data included 1,751,841 patients registered with 314 medical practices in Scotland and were analysed according to the number of conditions (from a list of 40 diagnoses – 32 physical and 8 mental) and by sex, age and socioeconomic status (measured from postcode). We found that multimorbidity was highly socially patterned, occurring more often and at an earlier age by 10–15 years, in those living in more deprived areas.

Figure 5.1 below shows the percentage of people in Scotland with two or more long-term conditions by age group and by deprivation. Multimorbidity increases with age for everyone, but in the deprived areas there is more of it, and at a much younger age. As can be seen from the graph, below the age of 85, the effect of deprivation on multimorbidity shows a perfect social gradient, with a shift to the left (meaning more multimorbidity at a younger age) for every decile of deprivation.

We found that it was unusual to have only one long-term condition. Most people had more than one. Figure 5.2 shows in each row the percentage of people with a single condition only (pale blue), those with the single condition and one, two or

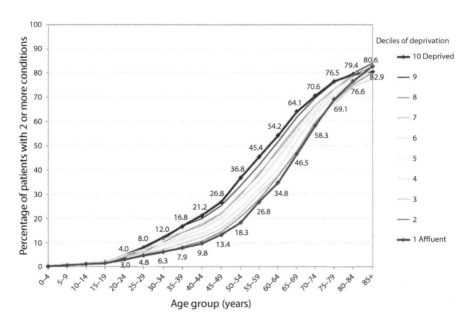

Figure 5.1 Prevalence of multimorbidity by age and socioeconomic status. (Reproduced from Barnett, B. et al., *Lancet*, 380, 37–43, 2012. With permission.)

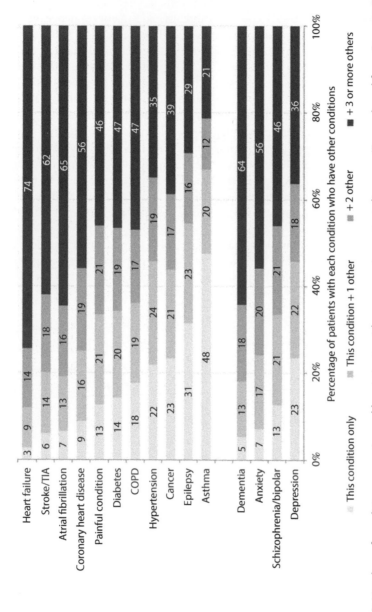

Figure 5.2 Number of conditions experienced by patients with common, important diseases. (Reproduced from Barnett, B. et al., Lancet, 380, 37–43, 2012. With permission.)

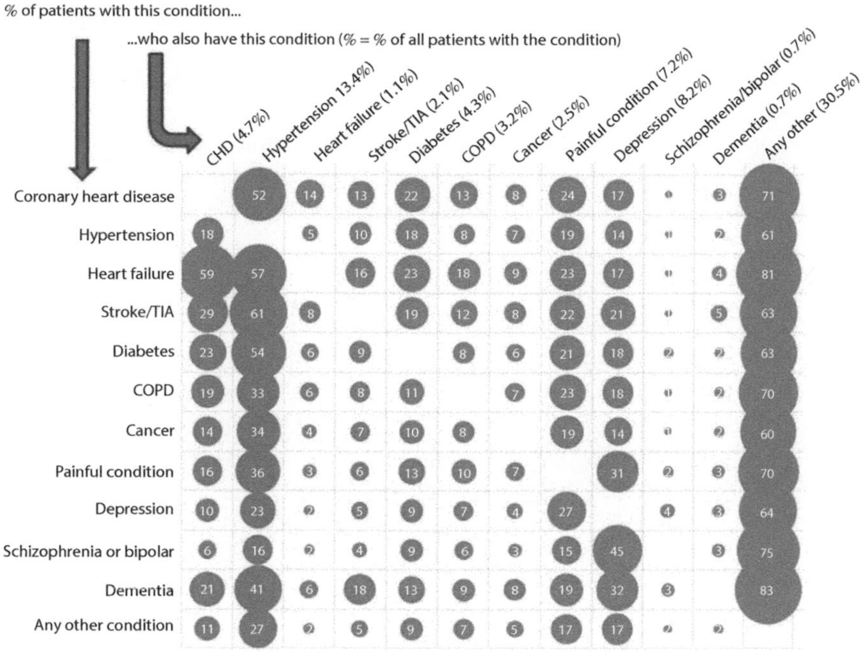

% of patients with this condition...

...who also have this condition (% = % of all patients with the condition)

	CHD (4.7%)	Hypertension 13.4%	Heart failure (1.1%)	Stroke/TIA (2.1%)	Diabetes (4.3%)	COPD (3.2%)	Cancer (2.5%)	Painful condition (7.2%)	Depression (8.2%)	Schizophrenia/bipolar (0.7%)	Dementia (0.7%)	Any other (30.5%)
Coronary heart disease		52	14	13	22	13	8	24	17		3	71
Hypertension	18		5	10	18	8	7	19	14			61
Heart failure	59	57		16	23	18	9	23	17		4	81
Stroke/TIA	29	61	8		19	12	8	22	21		5	63
Diabetes	23	54	6	9		8	6	21	18			63
COPD	19	33	6	8	11		7	23	18			70
Cancer	14	34	4	7	10	8		19	14			60
Painful condition	16	36	3	6	13	10	7		31			70
Depression	10	23		5	9	7	4	27		4		64
Schizophrenia or bipolar	6	16		4	9	6	3	15	45			75
Dementia	21	41	6	18	13	9	8	19	32	3		83
Any other condition	11	27		5	9	7	5	17	17			

Figure 5.3 Selected comorbidities in people with four common, important disorders in the most affluent and most deprived deciles. (Reproduced from Barnett, B. et al., *Lancet*, 380, 37–43, 2012. With permission.)

three or more other conditions (dark blue). Out of the 40 conditions we examined, there were none which had a majority of people with that condition alone. Most patients had multimorbidity.

Figure 5.3 shows for each common chronic condition the percentage of patients with different types of comorbidities. Concordant multimorbidity, on the left of the figure, shows the clustering of similar conditions, while discordant multimorbidity, on the right, shows the clustering of very different conditions such as depression and pain.

5.3 THE CHALLENGES OF MULTIMORBIDITY

When sorrows come they come not single spies, but in battalions

Shakespeare
Hamlet

*Health care systems will continue in the future to deal with emergencies, provide access to specialist investigations and treatments, give children a good start

* Parts of the following text appeared previously in an essay in the *British Journal of General Practice*. Watt G. The subversive challenges of multimorbidity. *British Journal of General Practice* 2015. doi:10.3399/bjgp17X691289.

in life and help people to die with dignity and in comfort but, increasingly and especially in developed societies, their major role will be to help people live longer and better in the community as they acquire more and more health problems in the second half of their lives.

Multimorbidity is not a new problem to be dealt with in old ways but a huge challenge to the nature, organisation, resourcing and culture of health care.

5.3.1 Defining multimorbidity

Epidemiology often reveals important insights by applying simple definitions and measurements to large numbers of people so that they can be studied in groups. A common approach is to define multimorbidity as having two or more conditions. The landmark study described above used this approach to show that multimorbidity increased with age, with an onset 10–15 years earlier in socio-economically deprived areas (1). Although prevalence rose with age, the demographic shape of the population determined that most people in Scotland with multimorbidity were under 65 years of age.

Such observations are useful; however, in clinical practice, a definition based on two or more conditions can be of little consequence. The most common comorbidity in older people is hypertension so that only one other condition is required to meet the definition of multimorbidity. This case definition offers little new challenge to clinicians or to services.

On the other hand, the most common comorbidity in deprived areas is a mental health problem (1) whose combination with another condition is likely to complicate the care that patients need and receive.

More demanding definitions of multimorbidity – such as five or more conditions, the combination of a physical and psychological health problem, or three or more chronic conditions from different body systems – have lesser prevalences, but steeper social gradients, and present a significantly greater clinical challenge (2,3).

Even so, many patients with multiple conditions are not 'complex', whereas some patients with single conditions are very 'complex'. Such distinctions draw on a wider body of knowledge, concerning not only the individual but also their circumstances.

5.3.2 Listen to the patient

For clinicians, the care of patients with multimorbidity can be complicated by multiple clinical targets and treatments (sometimes called 'polypharmacy'). While specific targets and treatments are usually evidence based, there is little evidence on how to combine multiple, and sometimes contradictory, treatments and targets in individual patients (4).

In such cases, an important source of evidence is the patient. Whereas Sir William Osler taught medical students *'Listen to your patient, he is telling you the diagnosis,'* today we *'Listen to the patient, she is telling you her treatment goals'*.

Professor Jan De Maeseneer from Ghent in Belgium (see Section 9.5), in his 2011 RCGP Mackenzie Lecture, described an elderly female patient with diabetes, heart disease, associated polypharmacy and other problems (5). Frequent encounters focusing on clinical management and treatment targets satisfied neither the patient nor the doctor. The turning point was sitting down to establish the patients' treatment goals which were a combination of function (e.g. being able to get out of the house or go shopping) and social participation (e.g. meeting with friends once or twice a week to play cards).

5.3.3 Patient experience

In life, as in the film, little happens in brief encounters. It is the serial encounter that matters, comprising all the contacts a patient has, some of which may be short and impersonal, but the most important of which involve long-term direction and common purpose, building patients' knowledge and confidence in living with their conditions and in accessing appropriate advice and support. Local health systems require not only this continuity and purpose but also the flexibility to accommodate starts, stops, restarts, diversions, events, successes, and disappointments (6).

The metaphor of a journey introduces the concept of destination and the criteria by which the journey may be considered a success.

When patients' serial encounters with health professionals are added up, what is being achieved and is it 'good enough'? Unlike the management of high blood pressure and similar conditions, where definition, measurement, audit and research are simple, there is no similar information system for longitudinal care and, in particular, the nature, extent and quality of care coordination (Section 5.4).

The 'treatment burden' comprises the work that patients must do to live successfully, understanding their conditions and medications, accessing services, and adapting their life and work accordingly (7). Too often the arrangement of services makes life more difficult for patients. George Bernard Shaw described all professions as conspiracies against the laity (8), not because they meet in secret to conspire against patients, but because of their tendency and ability to configure arrangements in ways that suit them.

Increasingly, the care of patients with multimorbidity involves a mixture of contacts with different professionals, services and resources. Such care needs to be composed, orchestrated and conducted to the patients' advantage (Section 3.7). However, the patient struggling to cope with dysfunctional, fragmented, local systems has become a commonplace (7).

5.3.4 Machines that do the work of two people

The comedian Spike Milligan described the invention of a machine that did the work of two men but required three men to work it (9). No health care system can afford such arrangements but, with the expansion of specialist services, this is the direction of travel.

Specialist services have diagnostic criteria or tickets of entry, assessment procedures to see if patients meet the criteria, waiting lists to control access, specific treatment protocols that are often evidence based and discharge back to other care when they are done. Of course, specialist investigation and treatment are important and are generally carried out to a high standard, but specialist clinics often leave a lot for generalists to do, for patients who do not meet the criteria, are not good at accessing services, have other conditions and who are not made better by specialist treatment.

A better balance is needed between the contributions of specialist and generalist care to health systems as a whole.

Extending Milligan's metaphor, the only affordable and sustainable future involves machines that do the work of two people, but which can be operated by one person. In practical terms, this involves small teams of health professionals working as generalists, unconditionally and consistently with patients they know.

With their patient contact, population coverage, continuity, flexibility, long-term relationships and trust, sometimes called the Essence of General Practice (10), general practices are the natural hubs of local health systems, but hubs on their own are insufficient. They need to be connected via spokes, or links, to a wide range of other resources and services. The NHS needs wheelwrights to build such local systems and, in particular, the relationships on which joint working depends (11). This is much more likely to be achieved by general practices reaching out than by external services trying to reach in.

The converse of practices looking outwards is that many specialist services would be more effective and equitable if they were linked more closely to general practices with their population contact, cumulative knowledge and generally positive relationships with patients. This book includes several examples of the benefit of embedding specialist and attached workers within practice teams (Section 7.1, Chapter 8, Section 14.2).

5.3.5 The worried doctor

The concepts of self-care and self-management imply the transfer of responsibility and agency from professionals to patients and have varied applicability depending on where patients are placed on the spectrum from 'worried well' to 'unworried unwell'. In deprived areas, such concepts are destinations rather than starting points. The treatment burden is increased, and life is made more difficult for patients having to access advice and support from multiple sources.

The patients who most need health literacy, confidence and agency in accessing multiple services for different conditions are least likely to have these attributes, especially when, as is common, their multimorbidity is complicated by a mental health condition (12). Such patients are easy to ignore and need a 'worried doctor,' or similar person, to steer their course, facilitate access, anticipate hazards and resolve problems (13).

Although most patients with multimorbidity are different from each other, their needs are frequently similar, comprising unconditional, personalised continuity of care. Specialist expertise and inputs may be required for diagnoses and treatments at key stages of the patient journey, but the continuing support that patients need is more likely to be generalist and local in nature.

5.3.6 Leadership

Three building programmes are required:

- Building strong patient narratives based on increasing knowledge and confidence in living with multiple conditions and making good use of available services.
- Building strong local health systems, based on general practice hubs, with referral links that are quick, local and familiar, whenever possible.
- Building links and collegiality between local health systems so that there is shared knowledge and consistency across primary care as a whole.

In the nineteenth century, Britain's industrial revolution was led not by scientists, inventors or investors, but by a cadre of entrepreneurs who knew how to combine knowledge, scientific inventions, raw materials and people in productive local systems. For the social revolution required to help people with multimorbidity live long and well in the community, similar leadership is required, to produce not goods and profits, but the multiple productive relationships, based on mutuality and trust, that make strong local health systems.

Health system development often depends more on building relationships than on re-structuring. In a King's Fund report, the active ingredients of coordinated care were described, including schemes for palliative care at home, mental health services, home care for people with dementia, care for older and frail people, and complex case management to reduce unnecessary hospital admissions (14). The report questioned the need for defined care packages, arguing that protocol-driven approaches lack the flexibility that patients with complex needs require. Such schemes are weaker without GP engagement, knowledge and leadership. Bottom-up approaches are needed to develop 'the building blocks of effective partnership working', rather than top-down approaches, no matter how well they may have worked elsewhere. Most of the projects took six to seven years to achieve the desired changes (14).

5.3.7 Information

The health information systems we rely on today all had to be imagined, developed, tested and refined before they could be used to audit and improve care. Two important new types of information are needed for integrated care.

First, primary care is a compendium of individual patient stories. Each is the product of serial encounters, involving all the contacts a patient has with services. Whether the story has a good ending depends partly on professional expertise, but also on patient enablement and the extent to which patients and professionals are concentrating on the same goals. If the patient narrative is the unit of currency, is the currency weak or strong? Can we imagine ways of collecting and using such information?

Second, the social capital within a local health system is simply the sum of the relationships within it and the uses to which they are put. Local health systems can be resource-rich but people-poor, or resource-poor and people-rich. What mechanisms do we have for assessing such social capital, to know whether the system is rich or poor, to support and reward the good and to weed out the bad?

5.3.8 Conclusion

Multimorbidity is a huge challenge to existing institutions, professional authority and ways of working. The knowledge and expertise produced by medical schools, mainly supporting the specialist paradigm, is not the type of knowledge or expertise needed to address complex multimorbidity, or the clinical leadership needed to develop local health systems. The dominant paradigm breaks problems down into their component parts. The new paradigm is about building, whether patient narratives or the relationships required to develop sustainable local health systems based on productive working across boundaries.

5.4 ASSESSING THE QUALITY OF GENERALIST CLINICAL CARE

KEN McLEAN

Assessing the quality of care that a GP or practice provides is a challenge. Most GPs and patients can recognise good care but teasing out the reasons for that feeling is difficult.

What is considered to be good care changes over time. Behaviours which were at one time considered innovative become normal practice or no longer relevant. For example, the Royal College of General Practitioners (RCGP) ran the Quality Practice Award (QPA) from the late 1990s until 2015. The award was achieved if over a hundred criteria were met and after a successful assessment visit. The award recognised what was considered to be the provision of the highest level of care. Criteria were amended annually as general practice improved. Version three in 1999 had criteria which asked for the management plans for at least seven major clinical conditions and audits of these. The subsequent introduction of the Quality and Outcomes framework meant that the vast majority of practices easily achieved this. In the same version, there was a criterion which asked for up-to-date textbooks and CD-ROMs which is clearly out of date now. QPA was stopped by the RCGP as, although it improved the care of patients in participating practices, it did not impact more widely on the care provided by non-participating practices.

Any assessment of the quality of care provided by a service is usually covered by one of or a combination of three factors; metrics, the customers' views and comparing performance against a set of standards or criteria set by 'wise men'. However, Quality Assessment is only part of the quality of care agenda.

The Juran trilogy classifies quality as consisting of Quality Planning, Quality Improvement and Quality Assessment.

The use of metrics to assess the quality of GP care has been flawed by the Quality and Outcomes Framework which only measures quality of care in a small percentage of the consultations carried out by GPs and practice nurses. The linkage to practice income has allowed a disproportionate effort to be focussed on single disease management. The problem at present is that the research to provide meaningful standards for multimorbidity care is not yet available.

Standard setting for practices by 'wise men' has been present in a variety of assessment systems since the 1990s. As well as the aforementioned RCGP QPA, the RCGP in Scotland ran a Practice Accreditation award from 2000 to 2004 and the RCGP ran an English version which became redundant when the Care Quality Commission standards became compulsory. Accreditation systems have also been used in Wales and Northern Ireland as well as some Commonwealth countries. There are problems with these systems. They are costly to administer and require significant resource input from practices which can be better spent on frontline patient care. The standards also tend not to be flexible enough to determine good clinical care for patients in all practices.

For example, same-day access to a GP may be more important to patients in a practice where there is a high number of unemployed people, whereas the availability of planned early or late appointments is valued more by patients in a practice with a high number of commuters. These systems also tend to focus on the care provided by the individual clinician or practice. They do not reflect the quality of care provided across the wider health and social care systems which are so relevant to those with several conditions. Nor do they tackle the interface problems between general practice and hospitals, social work and other primary care providers, such as community pharmacists. In recent years, the RCGP has moved away from a quality assessment stance to one focussing on quality improvement.

The Scottish approach to making quality standards more relevant has been to set up local GP clusters that decide their own areas that need improvement, set their own standards and measure their performance against these. It is too early to know if this approach will be successful; however elsewhere in Europe, quality circles have been shown to improve patient outcomes. The inherent localism is both a good and bad thing. It allows local issues to be prioritised but can also create situations where practices calibrate against each other and accept a lower standard of performance than other areas provide.

We are left with the patient view as a measure of the quality of care. It is, after all, their lived experience of their health that matters. Seeking patients' views on the quality of care can be done at individual clinician or practice level through questionnaires, the use of focus groups or patient participation groups. Until there is evidence on how we measure generalist clinical care in a multimorbid world, the patient voice will remain the most important component of any assessment.

As a start, practices may wish to collate the views of their patients on how their care measures against Starfield's four 'Cs': contacting (or accessibility), continuity, comprehensiveness and coordination. Such an approach would give a framework for assessing performance that is relevant to their own patients and help identify areas for improvement.

Finally, the RCGP has recently acknowledged that any strategy to improve the quality of care must take into account the quality of experience of the professionals providing that care. Demoralised and burnt out doctors and nurses do not provide the best of care for their patients.

5.5 COMPETING FOR POWER AND RESOURCE

It must be considered that there is nothing more difficult to carry out nor more doubtful of success nor dangerous to handle than to initiate a new order of things; for the reformer has enemies in all those who profit by the old order, and only lukewarm defenders in all those who would profit by the new order; this lukewarmness arising partly from the incredulity of mankind who does not truly believe in anything new until they have experience of it.

Nicolo Machiavelli
The Prince

Successive governments in Scotland and England have neglected generalist care, keeping funding and numbers of GPs steady while increasing funding and the numbers of specialists in both secondary and primary care by 50%. Increasingly, power and resource have been configured around managerialism and specialism, including specialisms in primary care, such as mental health and child health services.

Although the dominance of specialism over generalism in health care is ubiquitous throughout the world, reflections on UK experience may have wider relevance.

Support for hospitals is deep-wired in the public psyche. Threats to hospital services are guaranteed to generate public demonstrations. Politicians pledge their support for 'schools and hospitals' before other public services. As the place where most people are born, die, attend for major emergencies and are treated for serious conditions, this is hardly surprising.

Concentrating expertise and resources in hospitals is the sensible strategy, therefore, to provide the care that people need, on the few occasions that they need it, for everyone living in a local community. For the rarest diseases and most expensive investigations and treatments, additional centralisation is required via tertiary levels of care.

With centralisation goes specialisation, as described almost a century ago by Sir James Mackenzie (1).

We are all the creatures of circumstance, and our ideas are moulded by our experiences. Those employed in the study of medicine look at the subject in the light of their own experiences. As the subject is so large, one individual can have an experience of but a small part, so that there is no one capable of seeing it as a whole. The result is that medicine has to be studied in sections, and this leads to specialism. The authorities who guide and direct the progress of medicine are therefore men with but a limited experience and this leads to a limited outlook. In an attempt to bring together a body of men whose united experience, it might be thought, would cover the whole field, there is a danger that some section may be wanting, and thus a distorted view or a view lacking in perspective may be obtained.

The limitations of specialism are highlighted by multimorbidity. While on the one hand, hospitals can be models of efficiency in the handling of discrete episodes and the management of single conditions, weaknesses in continuity and coordination often result in patients having fragmented experiences and unsatisfactory outcomes, especially for elderly patients with multimorbidity.

The universal location of medical schools in tertiary centres of clinical excellence and the concentration of medical student education in such places has had unfortunate effects, as described by Lord Moran, Winston Churchill's doctor, in his evidence to the Review Body on Doctors' Remuneration in 1966 (2).

Chairman: It has been put to us by a good many people that the two branches of the professions, general practice and consultancy, are not senior or junior to one another but they are level. Do you agree with that?

Lord Moran: I say emphatically no. Could anything be more absurd? I was dean at St Mary's Hospital (medical school) for 25 years. ... All the people of outstanding merit, with a few exceptions, aimed to get on the staff. There was no other aim, and it was a ladder off which some of them fell. How can you say that the people who get to the top of the ladder are the same as the people who fall off it? It seems to me so ludicrous.

Chairman: But might not general practice be a vocation especially suited to those wishing to serve the community?

Lord Moran: If a man's vocation was obviously trying to help the community, would he not have more opportunities as a consultant?

Moran's views were soon considered old fashioned, but they linger on. In 2017, the Royal College of General Practitioners complained about the disparaging comments made about general practice by clinical consultants teaching in UK medical schools.

The political challenge is to establish a better balance between generalist and specialist care and, in doing so, to change the experiences of patients in practice and doctors in training. But power and resource are seldom given up by those who have them, and with most medical institutions being dominated by specialist views and with politicians, health managers and the media generally being in thrall to the medical establishment, shifting the health system's centre of gravity is not a simple task. We are at the beginning of a long process.

Rhetoric on its own is weak. Examples are needed of how general practice provides the health service with solutions to fragmented care, overuse of hospital services and widening health inequality, not only in individual general practices but by general practices working together as a whole system.

There are many barriers to developing this shared understanding.

- The perception of some opinion formers that much of the work of general practitioners is trivial, especially perhaps when their own experience of general practice is based on consulting with single conditions.
- The fact that the most important work of general practitioners, from the health service point of view, is with patients with complex multimorbidity, and is 'out of sight, out of mind'.
- The effect of generalist care is hard to document as it mainly results in non-events via the prevention, postponement or lessening of complications.
- The effects of a single general practice on population health and patients' uses of unscheduled care are difficult to demonstrate because of small numbers, the many sources of variation between practices and the lack of resource applied to this type of research.
- Over 90% of health research and academic funding supports specialisms, via biomedical and clinical research, for which multimorbidity, the bread and butter of general practice, is an exclusion criterion.
- The convention of grouping general practices for review and analysis by geographical area misses the information that could be obtained by grouping practices serving similar types of population (e.g. very deprived or rural areas) or with similar operating characteristics (e.g. practice size, type of premises).
- Most evidence-based medicine and associated clinical governance procedures are based on the management of single conditions, rather than the generalist approach required for multimorbidity. The Quality and Outcomes Framework (QOF) had good features but covered only 12% of consultations (3) and did not value or reward GPs for what good GPs are good at.
- The contractual independence of GPs keeps them at arm's length from NHS managers who are mostly involved in the management of hospital services and specialist services in the community.
- Central funders of health care do not trust the GP contract as a mechanism for investing in care where it is most needed, as there is no guarantee as to how increased funding will be spent.
- The contractual independence of general practices and the lack of infrastructure for shared learning lead to substantial variations in practice performance, often without practices being aware of it.
- Variation between general practices can result in the majority of practices being tarred by the behaviour of an aberrant few (e.g. high earning and/or high referring practices).
- Finally, the development and evaluation of 'community practice', based on general practices as natural hubs linked to other services and community resources, are at an early pioneering stage and are not ready for wholesale investment.

Whatever the relative importance and interplay of these factors, neither specialists and managers nor the politicians and civil servants they influence have tended to see general practice as an important or manageable solution to the problems commanding their attention. Affirmations of the importance of primary care are commonplace, but seldom matched by commensurate shifts in resources. As Margaret Mead observed

> What people say, what people do and what people say they do are three different things.

A different narrative is needed to compete for power and resource by providing better solutions for health service problems, such as multimorbidity, fragmented care, unfair treatment burdens, pressures on emergency departments, resource constraints, widening health inequality.

5.6 MAINTAINING SUFFICIENT NUMBERS OF CLINICAL GENERALISTS

Achieving the exceptional potential of general practice will only happen if there are sufficient numbers of general practitioners who are enthused, energised and supported in their work.

Recruitment at the outset of careers and retention towards the end of careers are important indicators of the attraction and satisfaction of working as a generalist clinician in the community.

Both are under threat, at least in the United Kingdom, as a result of pressures which detract from the intrinsic privilege and satisfaction of helping patients in need, especially over the long term.

The increasing needs of elderly patients, staff shortages, the demands of evidence-based medicine, the unfettered transfer of work from secondary to primary care and increases in electronically generated administrative work have conspired to lengthen and pressurise the working day. This is not an attractive prospect for potential recruits, especially when they have young families and wish to spend their evenings at home.

It is axiomatic that the challenges of recruitment and retention will only be solved if doctors see the prospect of a reasonable working day. Remuneration needs to be fair, both within general practice and compared with careers in medical specialities, but otherwise is not a main motivating factor (e.g. never once having been mentioned as an issue in the eight years of the Deep End Project).

More important determinants of professional satisfaction, energy and morale are autonomy, mastery and purpose (1).

Autonomy means the ability to make local decisions about how care is organised, within national frameworks of service delivery. Given particular local circumstances (e.g. history, geography, economy, staff, relationships, premises, etc.) the best local arrangements are unknowable at the centre and can only be developed on the basis of local knowledge, experience and accountability. Strong leadership is needed not only at the centre to provide the necessary support systems, but also at a local level to develop and maintain the most appropriate local arrangements.

Mastery concerns the many components of generalist clinical care, especially the management of complex multimorbidity, longitudinal care and the tolerance of uncertainty. Despite its importance to the health service as a whole and to the balance of care between scheduled and unscheduled (i.e. emergency) services, such work is often 'off the radar' of central management and specialist services. A cultural shift is required which values, supports and rewards what clinical generalists are good at i.e. providing unconditional, personalised and coordinated continuity of care. Mastery also needs to be developed in new leadership roles (Section 5.3).

Purpose implies a direction of travel from where we are to where we would like to be, broadening and lengthening the nature of care, strengthening local health systems and improving outcomes for patients. Such a purpose is denied to the casual doctor, earning a living via multiple locum or short-term appointments. Common purpose is a powerful and necessary force, if 'the best anywhere is to become the standard everywhere', but needs the commitment to, and infrastructure for, shared learning, without which there can be no shared responsibility.

Workload pressures can be reduced by enhancing the roles of nursing, pharmacy and administrative colleagues (2). Such changes need to be evaluated broadly, including such issues as the management of risk and impacts on continuity, coordination and coverage (i.e. what has been called 'general practice impact assessment').

In the Scottish Deep End Projects (Sections 7.1 and 7.2), which have applied the principles of autonomy, mastery and common purpose to primary care development, several features have been found anecdotally to aid both GP recruitment and retention.

- Adding a small amount of **clinical capacity** (about 10%) to reduce workload pressures and improve practitioner morale
- **Protected time**, of about one session per week, to release the time of practitioners so that they can apply their knowledge and experience to complex patients and to professional and practice development
- The employment of young practitioners in **GP Fellow posts**, partly to provide additional clinical capacity and protected time for host GPs, but supported academically and practically so that they are also involved in service development
- A **collegiate working environment** to share experience and learning within and between practices and with other professions and services

In this way, partnerships of experienced, inexperienced and academic GPs are involved in joint working to determine their future. The best advertisements for recruiting and retaining GPs are examples of GPs enjoying their work.

5.7 THE INVERSE CARE LAW

Julian Tudor Hart first wrote about the Inverse Care Law in a *Lancet* essay in
1971 (1).

> The availability of good medical care tends to vary inversely with
> the need for it in the population served.

The original article was not a systematic review of available evidence but rather a
polemic against injustice in health care delivery. Twenty years after the introduction of the UK National Health Service, Hart's first target was the divisive influence of market forces. By hoodwinking the worried well and avoiding complex
cases, there is always money to be made in health care and a queue of commercial
interests keen to profit from the lucrative trade.

Aneurin Bevan, Minister of Health when the NHS was introduced, sought to
avoid the consequences of financial barriers in health care, arguing

> Illness is neither an indulgence for which people have to pay nor
> an offence for which they should be penalised but a misfortune the
> cost of which should be shared by the community (2).

In the aftermath of World War II, won by bravery abroad and solidarity at home,
there was a determination in the United Kingdom not to return to the unfair-
ness of pre-war society. Bevan's book *In Place of Fear* (3) described his purpose
in addressing not only the fear of ill health but also its financial consequences.
Subsequent generations in the United Kingdom have benefitted from the generosity of their parents and grandparents at that time.

The introduction of the NHS was a great step forward, but it provided equality
of access rather than equity of needs-based care. Access was rationed in the same
way that butter, milk, eggs and bacon were rationed in World War II – everyone
getting the same, via a generally flat distribution of funding. What happened
after gaining access varied according to how the service was resourced, provided
and used. Hart's paper described the mismatch between needs and resources in
deprived areas. Over 30 years later, Watt used the swimming pool analogy (hence,
the 'Deep End') to describe how practitioners in deprived areas still lacked the
resource, principally time, to get to the bottom of patients' problems (4).

Of course, the most important determinants of poor health, and of differences
in health between social groups, operate outside health care and begin early
in childhood. Health policy has caught up with this understanding, and there
are many initiatives to improve children's start in life. Such measures will take
decades before they influence adult health.

Views on the contribution of health care to improving population health
lack consensus. Public health orthodoxy still reflects the view, put forward by
Professor Tom McKeown in the 1970s, that health care is a minor determinant
of population health and contributed less than 10% of health improvement since
the start of the century (5). McKeown may have been correct, but he was looking

back over a time which largely preceded organised health care and the development of evidence-based medicine.

Since that time, beginning with randomised controlled trials of the drug treatment of tuberculosis, there has been a huge increase in the number of treatments for which there is gold standard evidence of effectiveness in altering the natural history of conditions in individual patients. The mass delivery of such care has the potential to improve population health. Conversely, if such care is delivered more effectively to some groups than others, organised health care has the potential to widen inequalities in health. Very few reports on inequalities in health have recognised the role of inequitable health care as a social determinant of health.

An important observation from the literature on randomised controlled trials is the health benefit to patients receiving well-organised health care when randomised to placebo interventions compared with patients receiving conventional care outside the research setting. Notwithstanding the likelihood that trial participants are generally healthier than random samples of patients, the observation encourages the hardly radical proposition that well organised care is more effective than poorly organised care. The null hypothesis that there is no difference between the outcome of such care and care which is partial, impersonal, poorly coordinated and lacking continuity is highly improbable.

While the main contribution of general practice to population health may be considered, therefore, as providing unconditional, personalised continuity of care for all patients, whatever problem or combination of problems they have, this role has hardly ever been recognised, analysed or supported in reports, policies and strategies on health improvement. Instead, the general practice has been exhorted and incentivised to deliver a range of population-based measures, including risk factor assessments and health checks of unproven value, without additional resource to address the new caseloads which have been established.

In 2015, a paper in the *British Journal of General Practice* reported that although premature mortality and multimorbidity increased more than two and half-fold across deciles of the Scottish population, from the most affluent to the most deprived decile, the distribution of funding per patient per annum was virtually flat, especially across the four most deprived deciles (Figure 5.4) (6). Consultation rates rose by 20% across the spectrum but, in the absence of needs-based funding, could only do so in deprived areas by patients having shorter consultation times and/or GPs working a longer day.

Other research (Section 3.4) has described the implications of the Inverse Care Law at the level of individual consultations which in deprived practices were shorter, had a higher prevalence of multimorbidity and social problems, had poorer short- and medium-term outcomes (especially for patients with mental health problems – the most common comorbidity in deprived areas) and after which practitioners reported higher levels of stress (6). A study of video consultations showed that while patients with multimorbidity in affluent areas received 25% additional consultation time, patients with similar conditions in deprived areas received only average consultation times (7).

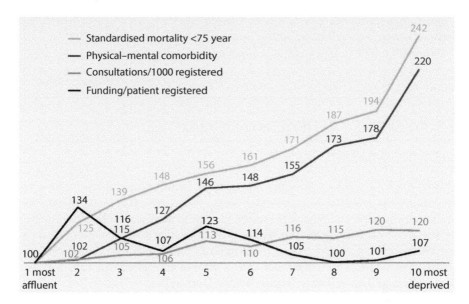

Figure 5.4 Premature mortality, complex multimorbidity, GP consultations and funding per patient per annum in deciles of the Scottish population. % Differences from least deprived decile for mortality, comorbidity, consultations and funding. Least deprived decile = 100. (Reproduced from McLean, G. et al., Br. J. Gen. Pract., 2015. With permission.)

The recently revised resource allocation formula for the new Scottish GP contract maintains the status quo with a 4% average increase in funding across the board from the most affluent to the most deprived practice populations (8).

These Scottish data have rung true for colleagues writing elsewhere in this book about general practice in deprived areas in Ireland, England and Wales (Sections 6.2, 6.3, 6.4 and 16.4). Over 40 years after first being described, the Inverse Care Law is still an endemic feature of general practice in the NHS.

For some time, colleagues involved in the Deep End Project thought that such facts would speak for themselves and lead to change, but the longevity of the Inverse Care Law has never been threatened by facts alone. Health systems are a compendium of competing interests with each interest defending its corner. To paraphrase George Orwell (9), the view that health care should have 'nothing to do with politics' is itself a political attitude, held mainly by those whose interests are being served.

In the United Kingdom, the Inverse Care Law is unlikely to be addressed by redistribution of existing budgets, especially when all parts of the system are underfunded. Unmet needs are easy to ignore, especially when health literacy, confidence and agency are low and other voices are louder. There is also the scepticism of politicians, health system managers and policy advisors about whether and how general practice can reduce health inequalities (Section 5.5). Advocacy has to be accompanied by examples of how health care improved, therefore, which is the theme of the rest of this book.

> He who would do good to another must do it minute particulars;
> General Good is the plea of the scoundrel, hypocrite and flatterer.
>
> **William Blake**

5.8 GP VIEWS ON HEALTH INEQUALITIES

BREANNON BABBEL

Efforts towards tackling Scotland's persistent health inequalities frequently emphasize the need to address wider social and economic factors (such as income inequality) (1). What has received less attention and exploration is the potential role of general practice. While general practice is not well positioned to prevent inequalities from occurring, unhindered access to culturally appropriate health care can slow the progression of the disease and reduce the effects of illness, thus helping to alleviate existing health inequalities.

The potential role of GPs in tackling health inequalities is linked to the inherent social responsibility within medicine, implying GPs have obligations not only to individual patients but also to the communities in which they practice. But how do GPs view these wider responsibilities and how do they view 'going the extra mile' to help their patients? These questions set the framework for a PhD research project, which involved conducting qualitative interviews with 24 GPs working in Scotland's most deprived practices during the autumn/winter of 2014–2015.

Given its concentration of deprivation, the majority of GP interviews took place within the Greater Glasgow and Clyde Health Board area. Fieldwork confirmed that a good way to get an overworked, overextended GP to talk at length was to bring them a cake. As a non-clinical 'outsider' from the US, bringing home-baked cookies to the interviews as a token of appreciation helped in building rapport with GPs.

The interviews revealed the potential for an advocacy role beyond traditional frontline work and clinical duties, harking back to nineteenth-century German physician Rudolf Virchow's description of physicians as 'natural advocates of the poor' (2). Views on this advocacy role varied, however, at individual, community and policy/political levels (Figure 5.5) (3).

5.8.1 Individual clinical care and social issues

> Your role is advocate. Your role is advocate with the hospital. Your role is advocate with the benefits agency.

Individual advocacy operated primarily in two ways – from a clinical perspective where symptoms are dealt with individually, or from a focus on social determinants of health. The latter meant dealing with the 'non-medical side of practising in a deprived area' by supporting patients beyond clinical care such as by writing letters in support of patients' benefits claims.

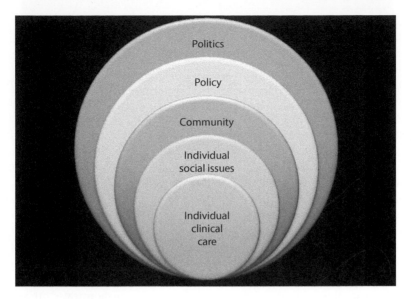

Figure 5.5 Hierarchical overview of GP 'Scope'.

5.8.2 Community

> I think we [as GPs] could do much more if we had a bit of time, better linking us up [with social services], and working together.

GPs acknowledged that medical illness is only part of the solution for patients in deprived areas. Another major part of the solution involves addressing social factors, which are often outside GPs' control, but which could potentially be addressed by strengthening connections with social services and resources within the communities they practice.

5.8.3 Policy and politics

> We don't have the resources to give people jobs or give people better housing, or more money, or deal with child poverty. That's a political issue and a social issue and we can only advise [on] what we see and what the effects of that is on patient's health ... But we should be part of the solution and part of the group of people who are designing strategy to help with all these problems.

As one GP noted, improving patients' housing and income levels were beyond the scope of general practice. Nonetheless, many GPs did feel they could provide a voice for the disadvantaged communities in which they work. Thus, GPs' professional scope shifts from simply advocating on behalf of individual patients to advocating on behalf of a patient population, working to influence policies impacting on their patients and taking a political stand. GPs subscribing to this belief felt they had the clout to provide evidence of the impact of social inequalities on health. The grouping of General Practitioners at the Deep End was seen as particularly helpful in providing a platform for this role (see Section 4.3).

One of the most important factors influencing what individual GPs felt they could accomplish at the higher levels of Figure 5.5 (i.e. underlying motivations for why they 'go the extra mile'), related to their views of patients, as expressed in terms of patient empathy, or willingness to 'walk in others' shoes', and how GPs discussed their patients. Demonstrating empathy meant showing a broader understanding of how patients' complex lives make behaviour change difficult. Considering patients living in deprived areas as 'deserving' of this support was significant in influencing a GP's commitment to improving living conditions and reducing wider structural inequalities.

When considering what could be done to address health inequalities, all GPs, regardless of their views about patients, held a common understanding around the importance of individual patient encounters. Specifically, they felt that encouraging health improvement strategies could mitigate negative social circumstances. Beyond individual encounters, however, it was primarily GPs who demonstrated greater levels of patient empathy who perceived their professional scope as extending to the higher levels of policies and politics (Figure 5.5). These GPs were more likely to identify structural causes of health inequalities and discuss personal obligations to use their own positions of power to advocate for local system and policy change.

In general, beyond the importance of empathy, GPs working in the 'Deep End' feel a social responsibility not only to address the clinical and social care needs of individual patients but also to influence the policies and politics that affect their patients' lives. Strained resources in the context of severe levels of multiple deprivation and multimorbidity make this professional and social responsibility difficult and has led many GPs to demand more resources for general practice in deprived areas.

REFERENCES

5.1 Confusing terminology

1. Hart JT. *A New Kind of Doctor: The General Practitioner's Part in the Health of the Community.* Merlin Press, London, UK, 1988. p. 100.

5.2 Multimorbidity

1. Barnett B, Mercer SW, Norbury M, Watt G, Wyke S, Guthrie B. The epidemiology of multimorbidity in a large cross-sectional dataset: Implications for health care, research and medical education. *Lancet* 2012;380:37–43.

5.3 The challenges of multimorbidity

1. Barnett B, Mercer SW, Norbury M, Watt G, Wyke S, Guthrie B. The epidemiology of multimorbidity in a large cross-sectional dataset:

Implications for healthcare, research and medical education. *Lancet* 2012;380:37–43.

2. McLean G, Guthrie B, Mercer SW, Watt GCM. General practice funding underpins the persistence of the Inverse Care Law: Cross-sectional study in Scotland. *British Journal of General Practice* 2015;65:e799-e805. doi:10.3399/bjgp15X687829.

3. Harrison C, Britt H, Miller G, Henderson J. Examining different measures of multimorbidity, using a large prospective cross-sectional study in Australian general practice. *BMJ Open* 2014;4(7):e004694.

4. McVicar R, Williamson AE, Cunningham DE, Watt G. What are the CPD needs of GPs working in areas of high deprivation? Report of a focus group meeting of 'GPs at the Deep End'. *Education for Primary Care* 2015;26:139–145.

5. De Maeseneer J, Boeckxstaens P. James Mackenzie Lecture 2011: Multimorbidity, goal oriented-care, and equity. *British Journal of General Practice* 2012. doi:10.3399/bjgp12X652553.

6. Watt G. The tortoise and the hare. *British Journal of General Practice* 2011. doi:10.3399/bjgp11X601415.

7. Mair F, May C. Thinking about the burden of treatment. *BMJ* 2014;349:g6680.

8. Shaw GB. *The Doctor's Dilemma*. Penguin, London, UK, 1946.

9. Milligan S. *Puckoon*. Penguin, London, UK, 1968.

10. Gillies J, Mercer S, Lyon A, Scott M, Watt G. Distilling the essence of general practice. *British Journal of General Practice* 2009;59:e167–e176.

11. Watt G. Inventing the wheel in general practice. *British Journal of General Practice* 2011;61:685.

12. Payne RA, Abel GA, Guthrie B, Mercer SW. The effect of physical multimorbidity, mental health conditions and socioeconomic deprivation on unplanned admissions to hospital: A retrospective cohort study. *CMAJ* 2013;185:E221–E228.

13. Watt G. Discretion is the better part of general practice. *British Journal of General Practice* 2015. doi:10.3399/bjgp15X685357.

14. Goodwin N, Sonola L, Thiel V, Kodner DL. Co-ordinated care for people with complex chronic conditions. Key lessons and markers for success. King's Fund, 2013. www.kingsfund.org.uk/sites//files//kf/field/field_publication/file/co-ordinated-care-for-people-with-complex-chronic-conditions-kingsfund-oct13.pdf.

5.5 Competing for power and resource

1. Mackenzie J. A defence of the thesis that 'the opportunities of the general practitioner are essential for the investigation of disease and the progress of medicine'. *British Medical Journal* 1921;1:797–804.

2. Review Body on Doctors' and Dentists' Remuneration (Danckwaerts Committee), Seventh Report, HMSO, 1966.

3. NHS National Services Scotland. Practice team information (PTI). Annual update (2012/13). Information Services Division, 29 October 2013.

http://www.isdscotland.org/Health-Topics/General-Practice/Publications/
2013-10-29/2013-10-29-PTI-Report.pdf.

5.6 Maintaining sufficient numbers of clinical generalists

1. Cochran J, Kenney C. *The Doctor Crisis. How Physicians Can, and Must, Lead the Way to Better Healthcare*. Public Affairs, New York, 2014.
2. Pink DH. *Drive. The Surprising Truth about What Motivates Us*. Canongate, Edinburgh, UK, 2011.

5.7 The Inverse Care Law

1. Hart JT. The Inverse Care Law. *Lancet* 1971;1:405–412.
2. Attributed to Bevan in Marshall TM in Social Policy in the Twentieth Century. Hutchison, London, UK, 1967 (but attempts to track down the original quotation have been elusive. See medium.com/@MarkleA/ something else Nye Bevan [probably] never said).
3. Bevan A. *In Place of Fear*. Heinemann, London, UK, 1952.
4. Watt G. The Inverse Care Law today. *Lancet* 2002;360:252–254.
5. McKeown T. *The Role of Medicine: Dream, Mirage or Nemesis?* The Nuffield Provincial Hospitals Trust, 1976.
6. McLean G, Guthrie B, Mercer SW, Watt GCM. General practice funding underpins the persistence of the Inverse Care Law: Cross-sectional study in Scotland. *British Journal of General Practice* 2015. doi:10.3399/bjgp15X687829.
7. Mercer SW, Watt GCM. The Inverse Care Law: Clinical primary care encounters in deprived and affluent areas of Scotland. *Annals of Family Medicine* 2007;5:503–510.
8. Mercer SW, Zhou Y, Humphris GM, McConnachie A, Bakhshi A, Bikker A, Higgins M, Little P, Fitzpatrick B, Watt GCM. Multimorbidity and socio-economic deprivation in primary care consultations. *Annals of Family Medicine* 2018;16:127–131. doi:10.1370/afm.2202.
9. Orwell G. *Why I Write*. Penguin Books, London, UK, 2004. p. 5.

5.8 GP views on health inequalities

1. McCartney G, Collins C, Mackenzie M. What (or who) causes health inequalities: Theories, evidence and implications? *Health Policy* 2013;113:221–227.
2. Virchow R. The aims of the journal 'Medical Reform.' In Rather L. Translator and Editor, *Collected Essays on Public Health and Epidemiology (1985)*. Science History Publications, Canton, MA, 1848.
3. Babbel B, Mackenzie M, Hastings A, Watt G. How do general practitioners understand health inequalities and do their professional roles offer scope for mitigation? Constructions derived from the Deep End of primary care. *Critical Public Health* 2017. doi:10.1080/09581596.2017.1418499.

6

Practices working together in the Deep End

The Deep End Project, comprising the collective activities of general practitioners at the Deep End, has spread from its origins in Scotland to similar projects in Ireland and Yorkshire/Humber and Greater Manchester in England. All are described in this section.

> Never doubt that a small group of thoughtful committed people can change the world; indeed, it is the only thing that ever has.
>
> **Margaret Mead**

6.1 GENERAL PRACTITIONERS AT THE DEEP END (www.gla.ac.uk/deepend)

In September 2009, RCGP Scotland helped fund an unprecedented meeting involving general practitioners from the 100 most deprived general practices in Scotland. It was the first time in the history of the NHS that this group had been convened or consulted (1).

The college had set up a working group to produce a report on what general practices in Scotland could do to address inequalities in health. The group made three early decisions. First, it would not replicate the many previous reports on inequalities in health, reviewing the partial literature and drawing partial conclusions. Second, it would not issue general practitioners with a 'toolkit', the approach of technocrats, which assumes that general practitioners only need to be told what to do. Third, it would listen to what general practitioners from the front line had to say. Without engagement with general practitioners, little else could be achieved.

The college established a budget which would allow locum fees to be paid. After some hesitation, the Scottish Government Health Department agreed to match the college's funding. On the day, GPs from 63 of the 100 most deprived general practices attended, along with 4 general practitioners from homeless practices in Glasgow and Edinburgh, 4 general practitioners from rural practices including small areas of deprivation and 2 civil servant observers. The day was spent talking in groups and open forums to capture the experience and views of general practitioners from the Deep End.

6.1.1 The Deep End

Practices had been ranked according to the proportion of the patients on their lists living in the most deprived 15% of data zones in Scotland i.e. groups of postcodes characterised by the Scottish Index of Multiple Deprivation (SIMD). Deep End practices have from 44 to 88% of their patients in this category, and collectively serve about a third of people living in the most deprived 15% of data zones. The other two-thirds are served by 700 other practices in Scotland. Thus, the Deep End Project has focused on blanket deprivation, rather than pocket deprivation, on the grounds that this is where a new start most needs to be made.

The Deep End epithet arose from the observation that while the prevalence of health problems rises 2.5–3.0 fold across tenths of the socioeconomic spectrum, the distribution of general practitioners is almost flat (Figure 5.4). In severely deprived areas, this results in a major mismatch of need and resource, with insufficient time to get to the bottom of patients' problems – hence the swimming pool analogy in which GPs at the Deep End are treading water. The analogy does not imply that general practitioners at the Shallow End are not busy, or that they do not have demanding patients, but their patients generally live much longer and mostly present less complex combinations of need.

6.1.2 The challenge

No one at the meeting was under any illusion about the many social determinants of poor health, and the need for measures outside general practice to protect and promote the current and future health of local populations. However, health care increasingly makes a difference to population health, especially in later life, and if this is delivered inequitably, health care can widen inequality. The challenge for health care is to find ways of increasing the volume, quality and consistency of care in deprived areas.

6.1.3 The practices

A total of 85 of the top 100 practices were based in Glasgow City, with 5 in Inverclyde, 5 in Edinburgh, 2 in Dundee, 2 in Ayrshire and 1 in Renfrewshire. 46 of the practices were based in two Community Health Partnerships (CHPs), in Glasgow East and North, where they comprised 84% of all practices. The other practices were a minority of practices in the CHPs in which they were based. Subsequent reclassifications of

SIMD changed the composition of the list of the 100 most deprived practices, with 85 practices appearing consistently and 35 appearing at one time or another.

The average list size in 2009 was 4,316, with 20 single-handed practices and 60 practices with three GP partners or less. There was no difference in the number of points achieved in the Quality and Outcomes Framework between Deep End practices and other practices in Scotland. About a half of practices were taking part in undergraduate teaching, a quarter in postgraduate training and two thirds in research (via the Scottish Primary Care Research Network) and primary care development (via the Scottish Primary Care Collaborative).

6.1.4 The meeting

The meeting was largely based on the sharing of experience and views. Many of the participants knew each other well from other activities. However, the focus on practices serving populations with concentrated deprivation and the absence of colleagues representing other types of practice were novel. In the final session, several commented on the almost immediate and strong group identity of practitioners from the 100 most deprived practices and the positive, cathartic nature of the meeting.

It was clear that Scotland does not have many of the problems of general practice in deprived inner-city areas, which have provided the context for much primary care development in England. Despite the heavy burden of health needs and demands, and their impact on both patients and staff, general practice serving areas of concentrated deprivation in Scotland is characterised by high quality (as measured by the QOF), high morale (as demonstrated by involvement in additional professional activities) and high commitment to improving services for patients (as evident by the discussions at the meeting). However, much more could be done.

The meeting strongly affirmed, indeed took for granted, the strengths of the general practice model, based on contact, coverage, continuity, coordination, flexibility, relationships, trust and leadership. There was frustration, however, from lack of resource, lack of support, lack of identity and marginalisation within current NHS arrangements. A strong theme was the problematic and dysfunctional nature of many external relationships, including those with non-practice employed staff, local authority services and community health partnerships. Many practitioners regretted the devaluing of consultations, considered to be the heart of general practice, by the financial incentives of the GMS contract.

The topics selected by participants for discussion were a mixture of issues particular to deprived areas (e.g. mental health and addiction, patient empowerment, resource allocation and support for practitioners) and issues of relevance to all general practices (e.g. multi-professional working, relationships with secondary care, infrastructure and premises and relationships with CHPs).

A GP from Edinburgh commented, 'I was in groups made up entirely of non-Lothian GPs. What was striking was not only that we got on well, but also on how much convergence there was in terms of the problems we face. I was in the primary/secondary care group and virtually everything said by Glasgow GPs, I could have said about Edinburgh – to a surprising level of detail. That problems seem to be so very generic and uniform across the board hopefully means that there might be generic and uniform answers too'.

6.1.5 What next?

The immediate challenge was to build on the engagement, enthusiasm, ideas and precedent generated by this first meeting. Could the extraordinary nature of the meeting be made ordinary, so that the top 100 general practices become a more effective force for improving primary care?

6.1.6 The Deep End logo

The Deep End logo includes (Figure 6.1):

The Deep End of a swimming pool
Gradients, including the steep slope of need and the flat distribution of resource
A flag for rallying under
A thistle
A spurtle (a traditional Scottish stirring instrument)
A sunrise (not a sunset)

6.1.6.1 A BRIEF HISTORY OF THE DEEP END PROJECT

Eight years later, the achievements of the Deep End Project included (2):

- Increased identity, voice, profile, influence, camaraderie and collegiality for general practitioners serving the 100 most deprived general practice populations in Scotland
- Participation by 75% of Deep End practices
- A website with 32 Deep End Reports (3), conference proceedings, publications, media coverage and news (www.gla.ac.uk/deepend)

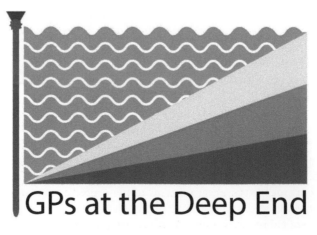

Figure 6.1 Logo of the Scottish Deep End Project.

- Advocacy concerning the nature and impact of the Inverse Care Law
- Affirmation that the principal contribution of general practice to addressing inequalities in health is via unconditional, personalised continuity of care for all patients, whatever problem or problems they present
- Dynamic collaborative projects including the Link Worker Programme (Chapter 8.1), Govan SHIP (Section 7.1), the Pioneer Scheme (Sections 7.2 and 16.7), attached alcohol nurses and embedded financial advisors (Section 14.2)
- Additional capacity for some Deep End practices including GP locums (Govan SHIP), GP fellows (Pioneer Scheme), protected time for GPs (SHIP and Pioneer Scheme), community link practitioners (promised for all Deep End practices from 2018), attached workers (SHIP, alcohol nurses, financial advisors)
- Productive partnership between service and academic general practitioners
- Parallel Deep End Projects in Ireland (Section 6.2), Yorkshire/Humber (Section 6.3), Manchester (Section 6.4) and Canberra, Australia

The main Scottish Deep End Projects and their key features are listed below. More information is available on the Deep End website (4).

6.1.7 Link worker programme (Chapter 8)

- Seven general practices hosted a full-time community link practitioner (CLP)
- Practice development funding
- Funded by the Scottish Government and administered via the Scottish Health and Social Care Alliance
- CLPs identified, developed and used links to community resources for health
- CLPs helped patients via signposting, one-to-one consultations, sorting problems and supporting referrals
- CLPs met weekly as a group for joint learning
- Strong central support including a programme manager and GP lead
- Independent evaluation by the Scottish School of Primary Care
- Programme now being rolled out across Scotland via 250 new CLP posts

6.1.8 Govan SHIP (Social and Health Integration Partnership) (Section 7.1)

- Four general practices have additional clinical capacity (about 10% extra) via GP locums
- Funded by the Scottish Government and supported by the Greater Glasgow and Clyde Health and Social Care Partnership South Sector
- Protected time for host GPs, used mostly for extended consultations with selected patients
- Initially attached social workers, then a new type of social care worker working preventatively below existing referral thresholds

- Two practices have attached community link practitioners (to be increased to four practices, as part of the national rollout of CLPs
- Monthly multidisciplinary team meetings (MDTs) in each practice
- Protected time for a GP lead
- Dedicated administrative and information support
- Independent qualitative evaluation by the University of Stirling
- Learning events to embed knowledge and develop a shared language across participating professional groups

6.1.9 Deep End GP Pioneer Scheme (Section 7.2)

- Five general practices have additional clinical capacity (about 10% extra) via GP fellows
- Funded by the Scottish Government and administered via the GGC Health and Social Care Partnership and RCGP Scotland
- Protected time for service developments by host GPs, including a lead GP role representing the practice in inter-practice and extra-practice activities
- Practice GP leads and GP fellows meet every six weeks as a group to share experience
- Regular day release sessions for GP fellows, with educational content and outcomes posted on Deep End website
- Shared learning among participating practices via online Trello platform and more widely via engagement with GP clusters
- Supporting recruitment of future GPs through engagement with medical students and the University of Glasgow REACH (widening access) programme
- Coordination via Lead GP and academic GP coordinator

6.1.10 Parkhead Financial Advisor Project (see Section 14.2)

- Two general practices have an embedded financial advisor, working as part of the practice team with weekly sessions in the practice
- Funded by the Wheatley Housing Group and Greater Glasgow and Clyde Health Board Health Improvement
- Facilitated and evaluated by Building Connections and the Glasgow Centre for Population Health
- New referrals, new claims and claimant incomes have increased (by an average of £7,000 per annum per claimant)
- The embedded advisor had access to information from medical records, with consent, and prepared draft letters for GPs to check and sign
- Ongoing internal evaluation and development via attached researcher
- Dedicated information support
- The project involved no additional work for the practice. GPs report that it released time for clinical issues
- The scheme is being rolled out in the local GP cluster of nine practices and evaluated by the Glasgow Centre for Population Health

6.1.11 Attached alcohol nurses

- Six general practices shared two FTE alcohol nurses
- Funded by Alcohol and Drug Partnership, Glasgow
- Specific evaluation not funded, used existing addictions resource to examine activity and outcomes
- Despite widespread support from all stakeholders and evidence of some positive outcomes, the pilot was not continued, due to addiction budget cuts and falling between service 'silos'
- A 'topic review' for a Health Technology Assessment by Health Improvement Scotland concluded that there is an evidence gap concerning the efficacy of attaching alcohol nurses to general practices in areas with high prevalence of alcohol use

In summary, the **10 active ingredients** of these primary care development projects include:

- Increased clinical capacity, about 10% extra, via GP fellows and locums
- Uses of extended consultations, mainly to coordinate uncoordinated care
- Protected time for GP leadership and service development
- Uses of link workers
- Experience of attached/embedded workers
- Multidisciplinary team meetings
- Advocacy for the 'unworried unwell'
- Practices working together in non-geographical clusters
- Dedicated leadership, coordination and support
- Shared learning events and knowledge dissemination

The **10 active ingredients** of the Deep End Project as a whole have been:

- Effective engagement with general practitioners, without which nothing else could happen
- A budget for clinical backfill, especially at the outset, to ensure representative participation (provided, initially, by the Glasgow Centre for Population Health, allowing flexible use of an underspent research grant)
- Identity, voice and common purpose i.e. the Deep End Manifesto (5), capturing GP's experience and views (Box 6.1)
- Reports and publications via the Deep End website (www.ga.ac.uk/deepend) and *British Journal of General Practice*
- Coordination and communication, mostly from an academic base
- Perseverance in preparing and waiting for opportunities to arise
- Responding quickly to opportunities for new meetings, collaborations and projects
- A programme of Deep End Projects giving expression and application to the Deep End Manifesto
- Working with academic colleagues to produce evidence of change
- Supportive partner organisations e.g. government (providing funding), RCGP Scotland (handling funds) and local NHS (facilitating projects)

> ### BOX 6.1: The six-point Deep End Manifesto (5)
>
> 1. Extra TIME for consultations
> 2. Best use of serial ENCOUNTERS
> 3. General practices as the NATURAL HUBS of local health systems
> 4. Better CONNECTIONS across the front line
> 5. Better SUPPORT for the front line
> 6. LEADERSHIP at different levels

The beating heart of the Deep End Project, however, has been its steering group, comprising 15–20 general practitioners, mainly but not exclusively from Glasgow, who have met over 50 times at evening meetings to share news, views, experience and plans. Steering group meetings prevented the project from being an academic exercise trying to influence general practice from the outside. They also provided continuity, solidarity and independence from existing institutions. Colleagues from Edinburgh gave the project a national dimension.

Academic GPs helped to coordinate and report Deep End activities. In this way, the partnership between academic and service GPs went much further than the usual academic/service collaborations for teaching and research. Both the Irish and Yorkshire/Humber Deep End Projects (Sections 6.2 and 6.3) have also involved academic input.

6.2 DEEP END IRELAND

SUSAN SMITH AND PATRICK O'DONNELL

www.deepend.ie

6.2.1 The Irish context

In Ireland, we have a public and private mix of funding for general practice. Approximately one-third of the population are entitled to free GP care and medicines with a copayment of €2.00 per item dispensed up to a maximum of €25 per month. This is called the General Medical Services (GMS) Scheme or the 'medical card' scheme. GPs receive an annual capitation payment based on the age of each of these medical card patients. There is no weighting for deprivation.

Patients who do not have a medical card must pay a consultation fee of approximately €50 per visit. All patients are entitled to free hospital care with some capped copayments for inpatient admissions. Free outpatient care is more attractive for patients who have to pay for GP care creating a perverse disincentive for GP management of common chronic conditions. Approximately 45% of people have private health insurance as this ensures timely access to diagnostic testing and specialist review in the private health system, compared to the public system, which has long waiting times.

Within this mixed public and private model, the Inverse Care Law applies to the most disadvantaged groups. Despite the fact that they have free GP care under the medical card system, they face long waiting times for diagnostic testing and secondary care services. Unlike more affluent patients, these patients generally do not have the means to pay out of pocket for tests and procedures. These delays result in later diagnoses and higher mortality from cancer in more disadvantaged areas in Ireland.

There are large variations in access to other vital clinical and social care services including child and adolescent mental health services, psychology, speech and language therapy and social workers. Given that there is no deprivation weighting in GMS payments to GPs, these pressures are particularly felt in deprived areas where there is often a high staff turnover of allied health professionals due to the pressured nature of work in these areas.

Irish general practice is described as being at a crossroads, with major concerns about its future due to the imposition of emergency cuts to GMS payments of 38% during the recession. These cuts were implemented in the context of chronically underfunded GP and primary care services, with only about 3% of the Irish health budget going towards general practice. This reduction has led to major difficulties for all practices in providing the most basic of services. Many practices are finding it difficult to recruit new GPs, and this is seen particularly in deprived and rural areas. This is all against the background of increasing multimorbidity and the complexity associated with caring for an ageing population.

6.2.2 Deep End Ireland

Deep End Ireland (Figure 6.2) grew out of a series of informal meetings initially between GPs working in disadvantaged areas of Dublin. The group has now expanded to include GPs from across the country. The primary aim of the group was to share experiences and ideas on how to manage the demands of work in these areas. We became aware of the Deep End Group in Scotland, and one of our

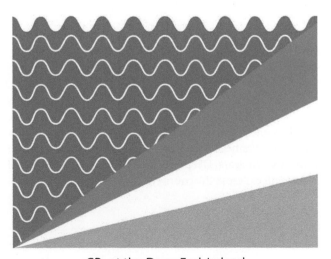

GPs at the Deep End, Ireland

Figure 6.2 Logo of Deep End Ireland.

members described herself as feeling like a patient who had finally found her support group. We then contacted the Scottish group in order to learn from their experience.

The first challenge we faced was trying to identify relevant practices in Ireland. Without universal patient registration or an existing deprivation payment, we have had to rely on multiple approaches, including geo-coding of practices and linking them to national deprivation data at district electoral division level. At the same time, we attended national GP meetings and publicised the group, inviting interested GPs to join.

Our first formal meeting was in 2012 when Dr Petra Sambale from Deep End Scotland came over to speak. Deep End Ireland has grown slowly since then with regular group meetings that have a planning and educational component, focusing on issues relevant to Deep End practice. We have also engaged with the Irish College of General Practitioners (ICGP) who have produced a report on the challenges faced by GPs working in areas of deprivation.

Over the years, we have engaged in multiple advocacy activities including meeting politicians, policymakers and medical organisations. Our 2016 national meeting was attended by about 70 GPs who agreed on the planned structure and aims of Deep End Ireland. This meeting led to the publication of the Deep End Ireland Report in 2017, in which we set out four key recommendations:

1. Fully functioning **primary care teams** in disadvantaged areas.
2. Strong **primary care infrastructure** in deprived areas that can act as hubs and facilitate linkage with community services and forums.
3. GP supports including **more consultation time** to address complex health needs; which could be facilitated through deprivation weighted capitation payments in a new GP contract and other options such as salaried GPs (working within GMS practices) and additional practice nurses or administrative staff.
4. Improved access to **diagnostics and other secondary care supports**.

These recommendations are based on the recognition that general practice has the potential to address health inequalities if adequately supported. They were presented to an All-Party Committee on the Future of Healthcare in 2016 that was established by the government in order to agree on reforms of the Irish health care system. The resulting Slaintecare Report emphasised the need for universal health care, free at the point of delivery and based on health need. The report referenced the Inverse Care Law and Deep End Ireland. However, the implementation of this report will depend on the negotiation of a new GP contract, a process that has been ongoing for over 20 years. Deep End Ireland now has over 93 GP members representing 85 practices across the country.

6.2.3 The future

While Irish general practice has been described as 'being in crisis' there are some positives. Most importantly, patients continue to report high levels of satisfaction and trust with GPs. There have been improvements in the structure and delivery of out of hours care through the cooperative systems, with benefits for both patients and GPs. There have been some minor developments in Chronic Disease Management programmes, though these only cover medical card patients. There are also examples of successful projects in disadvantaged areas that focus on addressing health inequalities, for example, a practice-based social prescribing initiative in Dublin. GPs remain eager to do more but struggle to deliver even reactive care in the context of financial cuts and recruitment challenges.

Generalism remains a fundamental attribute of Irish general practice. However, without the provision of sufficient resources to allow the general practice to adequately address the increasingly complex health needs of patients particularly in disadvantaged areas, the full potential of a generalist approach will not be realised. There is a glimmer of hope on the horizon, as a new GP contract is currently being negotiated and Deep End Ireland has been at the heart of attempts to incorporate contractual supports that will address the challenge of delivering high-quality care in disadvantaged areas.

6.3 GENERAL PRACTICE AT THE DEEP END IN YORKSHIRE AND HUMBER

TOM RATCLIFFE, ELIZABETH WALTON, BENJAMIN JACKSON AND DOMINIC PATTERSON

https://yorkshiredeependgp.org/

6.3.1 Background

General practice in areas of socioeconomic deprivation is a tough call (1). With many Yorkshire and Humber communities affected by post-industrial decline, GPs in our region see the stark reality of poverty on a daily basis, particularly when working in coastal areas and the major urban centres of Bradford, Hull, Leeds and Sheffield. The greater prevalence of multimorbidity (2), higher consultation rates (perhaps up to 20% greater than the most affluent areas) (3), encounters centred on complex psychological issues and trauma (4–7) and often limited support for patients with social problems (8) create intense and sustained pressure.

Whilst burnout is more common among GPs working in deprived areas (9) and resources are more stretched, we have found that there are incredible passion and commitment among these clinicians. Bring them together and you have an atmosphere crackling with excitement, innovative ideas and a genuine sense of hope and optimism that they can make things better for their patients in small but important ways.

In 2015, a group of postgraduate and undergraduate educators, all of whom work as GPs in deprived settings, set up General Practice at the Deep End Yorkshire and Humber (Figure 6.3). Inspired by the Scottish Deep End GP Project, the aim of the network is to tap into this desire for change and help tackle the region's stark and worsening health inequalities.

The group's core objectives were set out following vibrant meetings in October 2015 and March 2016, which have brought together 79 frontline clinical staff from across the region. As with the Scottish Deep End group, we targeted primary care staff working with the 100 most deprived GP practice populations in Yorkshire

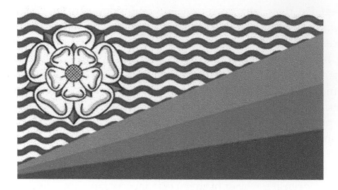

Figure 6.3 Logo of the Yorkshire/Humber Deep End Project.

and Humber. There was a consensus among frontline GPs that the group should tackle the challenges in four key areas:

- Workforce
- Education and training
- Advocacy
- Research

We have used the WEAR acronym to remind us of these areas of focus, which we agreed were the right places to start if we are to achieve long-lasting systemic change.

6.3.2 Workforce

Based on an audit of GP postgraduate training capacity in primary care, we found we had our own 'Inverse Care Law' operating across the region. 27% of Deep End practices are involved in training compared with 34% of practices in non-Deep End areas. Regionally, few areas bucked the trend. We concluded that this situation, if left unchanged, is likely to compound the shortfall in GP numbers in areas of high deprivation, where national data indicates there are fewer GPs per capita and a larger proportion of older GPs nearing retirement (10,11).

We have set about providing incentives and a streamlined GP trainer approval process for practices in the poorest communities. We have also attempted to build links between training and non-training practices and lobbied commissioners for equitable funding that reflects the greater health care needs in areas of deprivation. Members of the Deep End group have been instrumental in bringing new entrants, such as Physicians Associates, into primary care whilst advocating the need to maintain, expand and diversify the workforce in deprived areas as part of NHS England's GP Forward View plans (12). Finally, we look at setting up a 'Health Equity GP Trailblazer Scheme' to increase the number of salaried GPs working in deprived areas, which will subsidise GP posts in Deep End practices and fund time for these GPs to take part in service development and medical education work around health inequity.

The feedback from our symposia and study days has been very positive, with the sessions providing a substantial morale boost for sometimes tired and isolated Deep End GPs, who stated they value the opportunity to share learning and challenges with colleagues and form new relationships. It is hoped that our attempts to build a strong network and focus on education and training will improve recruitment, resilience and retention in Deep End settings.

6.3.3 Education and training

In 2016, we surveyed 103 GP Specialist Trainees at all stages of training in Yorkshire and Humber. The vast majority thought knowing about health inequity, multimorbidity and care of vulnerable groups is important for GPs. They identified the following specific learning needs:

- Understand the health problems affecting vulnerable groups
- Improve competence around communicating effectively with marginalised and vulnerable groups
- Understand the Inverse Care Law and its impact on health care delivery
- Increase awareness of local community groups working to tackle health inequalities
- Understand the role of GPs in policy formation/commissioning/public health relating to health inequity
- Understand the UK social security and benefits system

Further qualitative work showed that GP trainees had an appetite for working in more socioeconomically deprived areas but felt they needed help in acquiring the necessary knowledge and skills to survive in these challenging posts.

Since 2016, we have held workshops for GP trainees across the region, covering most vocational training schemes in Yorkshire, the Humber and North Lincolnshire. This has been backed up by the 'FairHealth' initiative, which aims to reduce health inequalities through educating health care professionals to help tackle health inequalities. FairHealth provides resources, online learning modules and patient narratives to help health care professionals understand the social determinants of health in the context of peoples' lives. We are coordinating a programme of postgraduate medical education, including study days and social accountability placements with the community and voluntary services, to ensure that every GP coming through our region's postgraduate programmes receives training around tackling health inequity. This is underpinned by a 2017 Delphi study that helped us define a 'Curriculum for Health Inequity', the full text of which is available on the www.fairhealth.org.uk website.

At undergraduate level, the Deep End group have been excited by Sheffield University's recently launched and popular social accountability placement for students. The university has also approved the appointment of a clinical teaching fellow to support the expansion of current undergraduate placements in more deprived areas. The development of a clinical Deep End student-selected module teaching is being underpinned by a national survey of health inequity teaching during GP placements in medical schools and feedback from patients and GPs working in Deep End practices.

For established and recently qualified GPs, we are creating three geographical professional development hubs in South Yorkshire, West Yorkshire and Hull/North Lincolnshire and East Yorkshire Coast. We are hosting regular local meetings for GPs, who define their own CPD programme. Our blog (www.york shiredeependgp.org) and annual meetings, which initially spanned Yorkshire and Humber and, in 2017, also incorporated GPs from Greater Manchester, have created a face-to-face and online network that offers support to GPs operating under huge pressure at the Deep End.

6.3.4 Advocacy

Michael Marmot and his colleagues implore us to 'rise up against the organisation of misery' (13). GPs are respected and often articulate members of the community and well placed to represent the needs and interests of their patients. Whilst there are challenges in finding the time to work as advocates for our communities alongside a busy day job, we have provided materials to support GPs in this role, including a summary of evidence around the Inverse Care Law for funding and workforce in general practice regionally and nationally, as well as training sessions on medical advocacy. Our members have raised the issue of health inequity at local and regional levels among senior commissioners and policymakers to ensure it remains a priority within the emerging NHS structures (14).

A number of members of the group have been involved in social prescribing and psychiatric liaison/well-being schemes that are attempting to shift care for patients with primarily psychosocial problems away from a traditional medical model designed to deal with physical health complaints. This approach has been promoted to commissioners across the region and is steadily gaining traction.

6.3.5 Research

On the research side, members of the network have been instrumental in setting up a Deep End Research Cluster starting in Sheffield and funded by the NIHR Clinical Research Network. Nine practices from the most deprived areas of Sheffield are taking part to recruit and help shape research from our practices in the hope of improving care for our patients, who have been consulted via an active patient participation network. A Delphi study is about to be launched to clarify where research and policy should focus to tackle health inequalities.

During our symposia, Deep End GPs have asked us to:

- Investigate barriers to self-care, access and uptake of preventative services at the Deep End
- Provide help with evaluating and describing new initiatives/service (e.g. interpreting services, social prescribing, proactive case management and care for patients with dual substance misuse and mental health diagnoses)
- Compile and share a regular synopsis of research relevant to Deep End GPs that can be easily accessed and used by frontline GPs

Across the region, there is a great deal of relevant academic activity, which we are attempting to share and publicise through our networks. Members of our network have undertaken two research projects with medical students at Leeds University. The first analysed attitudes of GP specialist trainees to working in areas of high deprivation (see above) and the second examined GP workforce distribution, finding that there were fewer GPs per capita in the region's most deprived areas. At Sheffield University, network members have been involved in research into resilience strategies among GPs working in areas of high socioeconomic deprivation, which has found that flexibility, adaptability and a team-based approach are essential in fostering integration of personal and professional values that protect practitioners (15). Another project has focussed on self-care in patients with COPD living in Deep End areas. This found that a psychological impact of the condition is key to self-management and is often overlooked in busy primary care consultations.

6.3.6 Where next?

The Deep End network cannot take credit for the work being done by incredibly dedicated and passionate clinicians across Yorkshire and Humber to try and address health inequity, but we have played a part in bringing colleagues closer together and raising the profile of Deep End general practice. We will continue to nurture and build this network, putting health inequity at the heart of postgraduate and undergraduate medical training and continuing to promote research and advocacy work that focuses on the needs of the poorest, most marginalised and vulnerable people in our region. Deep End general practice has extraordinary potential to improve lives, and we will play our part in making this happen.

6.4 DEEP END GREATER MANCHESTER

JOHN PATTERSON

https://www.sharedhealthfoundation.org.uk/deepend-gm

The NHS needs to be best where it is needed most. In practice, the opposite scenario is more likely. This injustice appears not to occur intentionally but rather out of the perfect storm of mismatched demand and resource. The Deep End movement is trying to highlight and understand why this storm blows and offer solutions to communities, workers and system leaders caught in the tempest. This is Greater Manchester's story.

Deep End Greater Manchester (GM) (Figure 6.4) started as a pragmatic practitioner and patient tale. Just as Tudor Hart saw the people first and then formulated his Inverse Care Law, we in North West England first saw the families affected by avoidable deaths under 65, households without any meaningful employment, children with treatable conditions in acute distress in A&E departments, excess use of painkillers, fragile mental health, schools struggling with attendance, increased polypharmacy, homelessness and hopelessness. As individuals and groups of practitioners, we have shared both anger at these injustices and compassion to seek their remedies.

The remedies are seldom simple. Sometimes, it is health care institutions that perpetuate the injustice. In GM, Deep End teams have found a 'Health Inequality

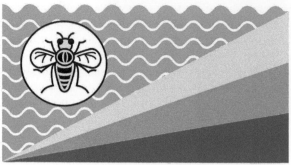

GPs at the Deep End GM

Figure 6.4 Logo of Deep End Greater Manchester.

Bubble'. In any primary care disease register, there exists a visible and rewarding group of patients whose care plan is working well (R, Figure 6.5). Across Manchester, there are just over 150,000 people whose diabetes is 'well controlled' yet this can mask those who are struggling to hit targets (M), to engage (E), or even to be diagnosed (U).

Although our computers light up green with clinical attainments, 51,000 people have no functioning care plan. Health inequality is created between the seen and the unseen. All the evidence indicates that people in this bubble are more likely to live in areas of social disadvantage. Our challenge is to find, diagnose, persuade and partner – in short, to see them.

From before the formation of the NHS, generations of health care practitioners have worked hard in the endemic deprivation of North West of England. What is new in the last few years is the use of 'Deep End' methodology to bring together many of these teams to form a supportive body of those who serve some of the hardest-pressed neighbourhoods in GM.

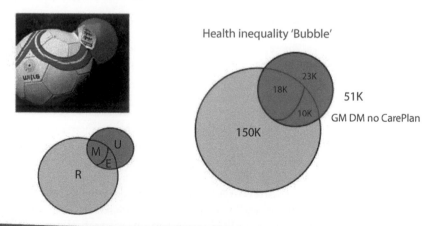

Figure 6.5 Numbers of well controlled, poorly controlled, unengaged and undiagnosed diabetic patients in Greater Manchester.

Together we intend to take on the challenges of primary care in our area, which are not unique but are heightened in the context of poverty. So far, we have shared best practice, facilitated research, increased resilience, explored new models and are starting to address workforce and training issues. We acknowledge all the good work that proceeds and accompanies us and lay no claim that 'Deep End' is the only effective way to address our shared issues.

Our recent journey began in 2009 when a young medical student (Now Dr Laura Neilson) made use of the then new Alternative Provider Medical Service (APMS) contract in general practice to form a community interest company (CIC) to provide primary care services to Fitton Hill estate in Oldham. Recognising the existence of the Inverse Care Law, we began rifling through the best evidence and case studies we could find. Most important, we needed:

- To focus on secondary prevention, especially finding and partnering with patients to help them gain control of their long-term conditions. Active case finding and a highly skilled nursing workforce would prove essential
- Longer appointments to recognise the earlier onset of multimorbidity
- To recruit people who lived in the communities of each practice as much as possible in terms of support staff
- To consider patients as members of interdependent households
- An in-house mental health service
- An additional worker and model to address the triad of (i) medical and social care complexity, (ii) engagement and motivational issues, (iii) the burden of poverty
- A culture of candour, kindness and continuous training of the workforce
- 'Community' as the preferred model of health care delivery whenever possible

In 2012, we attended a Health Inequality conference at Nuffield College Oxford and first met Graham Watt. Hearing about the emergence of the Deep End in Glasgow, both energised and reassured us that we were on the correct path. It was striking that it took an external locus such as the university there to bring together all the individual teams working so hard in deprivation and to equip the thinking and writing that had since emerged. It is a truism that those GPs working hardest, and successfully, in the highest disease-burdened areas are unfortunately often those least resourced to publish and share what they have learned. This changed with the advent of Deep End.

After several years of growing correspondence and encouragement from Glasgow, we were found by a social philanthropist in Manchester who had a pre-existing deep commitment to social justice and health inequality within the North West. His name is Michael Oglesby and through his charitable trust, a 'Shared Health Foundation CIC' was formed. Deep End GM sits within this as a funded project. The timing of this development coincided with the Manchester Devolution Act and the formation of the Greater Manchester Health and Social Care Partnership (GMHSCP).

The first Deep End Greater Manchester (GM) conference was held in September 2016 at the re-purposed Gorton Monastery. Over 100 doctors, nurses and students attended. An open invitation was advertised 'to all who considered themselves working in deprivation.' Like our Scottish forebears, we invited the 100 practices whose populations made up the most hard-pressed neighbourhoods. In September 2017, over 200 doctors of all grades, including students, attended a shared meeting with Deep End Yorkshire/Humber.

Between these yearly regional conferences, we aim to meet quarterly for planning and study days. As a group, we have decided to concentrate on workforce issues, education and training. Traditional GP speciality training has always been impressively broad. So far on these days, we have provided deeper training around mental health, self-resilience, motivation and engagement, substance abuse and approaches to 'medically unexplained symptoms,' to mention a few. Where possible we aim for the teaching to be provided by colleagues with specialist knowledge and experience from within the group.

The approaches we have taken towards workforce have been in partnership with the Manchester Medical School and GMHSCP. The joint aim is to provide an educational pathway from secondary school to postgraduate GP speciality training which focuses on recruiting practitioners from disadvantaged communities and preparing them to deliver sustained high-quality health care matched to the needs of those communities. It has been a pleasure to find the university already enacting far advanced plans along these lines. As of April 2018, we together provide several adapted or new options such as

- Short-term (four weeks) shadowing exposure to primary care in the Deep End as early as possible in the academic process.
- Short-term (four weeks) involvement in specific health inequality modules (such as health literacy) for year four and five students.
- A flagship 11-week deprivation and social care module with placements in thriving Deep End GP teams and parallel placements in third-sector organisations such as homeless shelters or drug and alcohol services. This scheme includes a regularly relevant taught syllabus provided by the best current practitioners we can find.
- In February 2019, we will admit our first year of post-foundation doctors to a new GP Specialty Trainee Programme based in the central and northeast regions of Greater Manchester. This will cover the usual RCGP syllabus with a strong focus on deprivation, inclusion health and self-care.

These four schemes have been made possible through a close partnership between the North West Deanery, Manchester Medical School, the Shared Health Foundation and regular GP teams working daily with the most hard-pressed households. It is also an example of Deep End groups supporting each other as we have received inestimable help from the North Dublin GP Training Programme (1) (Section 16.5). We have one Fellow in place to help with research and evaluation of this and other schemes.

The GMHSCP has been very supportive of the emergence of Deep End GM and has incorporated elements of Deep End GM into mainstream delivery. Our 'Focused care' model is a central part of the GMHSCP Population Health Plan, referred to as a 'New model of primary care for deprived communities' (2).

Focused Care provides an embedded worker, training resources and a practitioner community to GP practices with lists in the bottom quintile of deprivation. From April 2018, this scheme, funded between the central GMHSCP and local CCGs, is active in over 50 practices and has recruited over 1,000 households to active case management with practice teams. Large-scale evaluation is ongoing. Earlier results show high levels of patient and GP satisfaction, better health care utilisation (including 40% reductions in A&E use), plus increased uptake in preventative, public health and interventions for long-term conditions. The return on investment is projected to be between £2.5 and 3.5 for each £1 spent.

A key theme of the Deep End GM experience has been 'making the invisible visible.' This is true for the practitioners involved, and it has been a joy to watch colleagues realise that they are more skilled and more impactful than they had realised. Providing time and additional resources for overstretched colleagues to reflect and re-group has been one of the highlights of the project so far.

The most potent unveiling by Deep End GM, however, involves the discovery of households, often rendered 'invisible' to the services they need by our mutual problem of engaging with each other. We are starting to discover solutions. One day in the future, the lessons learned in Deep End groups will end up as mainstream health care behaviour and we will all be the beneficiaries of these gains at the margins.

REFERENCES

6.1 General practitioners at the Deep End (www.gla.ac.uk/deepend)

1. Deep End Report 1: General practitioners at the Deep End. September 2009. www.gla.ac.uk/deepend.
2. Deep End Report 32: 8 years of general practitioners at the Deep End. November 2017. www.gla.ac.uk/deepend.
3. Short summaries of meetings and activities (2010 to 2016). 2016. www.gla.ac.uk/deepend.
4. Deep End website at the University of Glasgow. www.gla.ac.uk/deepend.
5. Deep End Report 20. What can NHS Scotland do to prevent and reduce health inequalities? April 2013.

6.3 General practice at the Deep End in Yorkshire and Humber

1. O'Brien R, Wyke S, Guthrie B, Watt G, Mercer S. An 'endless struggle': A qualitative study of general practitioners' and practice nurses' experiences of managing multimorbidity in socio-economically deprived areas of Scotland. *Chronic illn.* 2011;7:45–59.
2. Barnett K, Mercer SW, Norbury M, Watt G, Wyke S, Guthrie B. Epidemiology of multimorbidity and implications for health care, research, and medical education: A cross-sectional study. *Lancet.* 2012;380 *Chronic Illn.*:37–43.

3. McLean G, Guthrie B, Mercer SW, Watt GCM. General practice funding underpins the persistence of the Inverse Care Law: Cross-sectional study in Scotland. *Br J Gen Pract.* 2015;65:e799–e805. doi:10.3399/bjgp15X687829.
4. Mercer SW, Watt GC. The Inverse Care Law: Clinical primary care encounters in deprived and affluent areas of Scotland. *Ann Fam Med.* 2007;5:503–510.
5. Mercer SW, Higgins M, Bikker AM, Fitzpatrick B, McConnachie A, Lloyd SM, Little P, Watt GCM. General practitioners' empathy and health outcomes: A prospective observational study of consultations in areas of high and low deprivation. *Ann Fam Med.* 2016;14:117–124.
6. Stirling AM, Wilson P, McConnachie A. Deprivation, psychological distress, and consultation length in general practice. *Br J Gen Pract.* 2001;51:456–460.
7. Watt G. General practitioners at the Deep End: The experience and views of general practitioners working in very deprived areas. *Occas Pap R Coll Gen Pract.* 2012;89(i–viii):1–40.
8. Hart JT. The Inverse Care Law. *Lancet.* 1971;297:405–412.
9. Pedersen AF, Vedsted P. Understanding the Inverse Care Law: A register and survey-based study of patient deprivation and burnout in general practice. *Int J Equity Health.* 2014;13:121.
10. Asaria M. Unequal socioeconomic distribution of the primary care workforce: Whole-population small area longitudinal study. *BMJ Open.* 2015;6:e008783. doi:10.1136/bmjopen-2015-008783.
11. National Audit Office. *Stocktake on Access to General Practice.* London, UK: National Audit Office, 2015, www.nao.org.uk.
12. NHS England. *GP Forward View.* London, UK: NHSE, 2016.
13. Marmot M, Allen J, Goldblatt P, Boyce T, McNeish D, Grady M, Geddes I. Fair society, healthy lives: *The Marmot Review.* 2010. *The Marmot Review,* 2014.
14. Jackson B, Irvine H, Walton E. General Practice and the Sustainability and Transformation imperatives. *Br J Gen Pract.* 2017;67(658):196–197.
15. Eley E, Jackson B, Burton C, Walton E. Professional resilience in GPs working in areas of socio-economic deprivation: A qualitative study. *Br J Gen Pract.* Accepted for publication May 2018.

6.4 Deep End Greater Manchester

1. The North Dublin City GP Training Programme. http://www.healthequity.ie/education-ndcgp.
2. The Greater Manchester Population Health Plan 2017–21, pp. 51–54. http://www.gmhsc.org.uk/assets/GM-Population-Health-Plan-Full-Plan.pdf.

7

Addressing the Inverse Care Law

GPs at the Deep End argue that the Inverse Care law is best understood as the difference between what they can do with the existing resources and what they could do if better resourced.

Two Deep End Projects, Govan SHIP and the GP Pioneer Scheme, have released the time of experienced GPs via protected sessions, which were made possible by the placement of young GPs in practices, either as long-term locums or as salaried GP fellows. The Pioneer Scheme also provides practices with additional clinical capacity.

The following accounts describe what can be achieved to address the Inverse Care Law with GP protected time.

7.1 THE GOVAN SHIP PROJECT

JOHN MONTGOMERY

The Govan SHIP (Social and Health Integration Partnership) was conceived in Govan Health Centre in Glasgow, a health centre hosting four Deep End practices, and went live in April 2015. The Scottish Government had introduced legislation to integrate health and social services. GPs in the health centre felt that if this policy was to succeed, it would need to be based on integrated working at the level of individual GP practices and individually aligned social workers.

They approached the local senior Community Health Partnership Director, the Director of Social Work and the Professor of General Practice to collaborate on a proposal, which was subsequently endorsed and funded by the Scottish Government. This cooperation between different specialties resulted in a significantly expanded remit involving integrated working with several other disciplines in addition to social work (Figure 7.1). Each practice would be resourced to employ a four session per week GP locum whose clinical contribution would give each GP principal one session per week of protected time.

This small amount of protected time for experienced GP principals allowed the development of new ways of working. Examples include the ability of GPs to have extended consultations, either in the practice or the patients' home, with

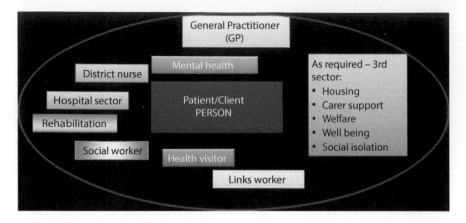

Figure 7.1 The Govan SHIP Project.

targeted complex multimorbid patients with significant health needs, which could not be met adequately in standard ten-minute consultations i.e. following the example of the Care Plus Study (1) (Section 3.4).

Attendance at social work case conferences involving vulnerable children and adults and closer working relationships with social work colleagues became possible as a result of the protected time. Polypharmacy reviews, preparation for multidisciplinary team (MDT) meetings and the development of informative electronic key information summaries (eKIS) were other examples. Further details of GPs' uses of extended consultations together with a sample of representative case studies can be found in Deep End Report 29 (www.gla.ac.uk/deepend).

Protected time also allowed GPs to engage in leadership activities, with virtually every participating GP responsible for leading on different and varied work streams:

- Lead clinician for SHIP
- Vulnerable children and families plus education
- IT
- Frail elderly
- Physiotherapy
- Pharmacy
- Mental health
- Unscheduled care
- Housing

In addition to the two full-time GP locums providing input to the four practices, other key additional resources included two fully qualified social workers, one covering vulnerable adults and the other covering vulnerable children and adults; a full-time project manager; and an administrative assistant to help with the logistics of MDT meetings. Two practices also had embedded community links practitioners (Section 8).

Our Project Manager describes his job description as being responsible for herding cats. His diplomatic skills were needed to help mould relationships between the different disciplines, especially at the beginning (2). Central to our integration agenda was the development of structured practice-based MDT meetings, taking place for two hours every month in each practice. A referral form was created for completion by any of the disciplines in advance of the meeting and also to record agreed outcomes as a result of MDT discussion.

Our project administrator arranged the dates and rooms for the MDT meetings, compiled the register of patients to be discussed (approximately 20–25, on average), circulated to all participants in advance and ensured that the necessary IT support was in place. A key aspect of MDT meetings is the ability of social work colleagues, community mental health workers, health visitors, district nurses and GPs to access their individual information systems during the course of the meeting. Although the systems themselves are not connected, being able to access each system at the meeting greatly facilitates the quick and efficient sharing of information and helps to ensure that a shared management plan is quickly constructed.

The meetings are organised in four sections: vulnerable children, families, adults and palliative care. If appropriate, an eKIS is then prepared with as wide a distribution as possible for all disciplines with access to it in order to maximise coordination of care and ensure that the patients' wishes are respected. The number of individuals attending MDT meetings and the time they spend in attendance varies, depending on the mix of cases, but GPs and the aligned social workers are generally present for the whole meeting.

7.1.1 Monitoring progress

Our administrative staff have been the key to ensure that we collect the data needed to monitor the consequences to patients of this team approach to patient care.

In terms of overall numbers, the SHIP practices had a combined population of some 14,200 patients with the targeted SHIP cohort comprising 899 patients (6.3% of the total).

We divided project patients, who were still registered at June 2017, into six-month tranches, based on their date of entry to the project, and looked at their GP interactions prior to and after SHIP involvement. GP utilisation was defined as all GP entries to the practice information system (EMIS) including telephone calls, approving lab results, home visits, in-surgery consultations, and so on.

Demand by these groups of targeted individuals had previously been higher than the practice average, had been increasing over time, peaked during the period of intervention and then reduced back towards original levels. It may be that some of these would have regressed back to the mean in any case. In such cases, the benefit from the project has been that early intervention accelerated this. Looking at the profile of these patients, they had significantly higher levels of multimorbidity in comparison to the baseline average for the practices using a developed project-specific tool – see the contribution by Brian Milmore below.

7.1.2 Overall GP demand and comparison with other practices

We compared data from a group of other practices in Glasgow with similar population size, demographics, deprivation and other characteristics (Figure 7.2). SHIP practices demonstrated a statistically significant decrease in all GP interactions during the time of the project whilst comparator practices showed a statistically significant increase. This was particularly striking when looking at home visiting rates, which declined at a significantly faster rate in SHIP practices compared with the comparator practices. Our interpretation is that taking a proactive approach to patients in greatest need decreases the requirement for crisis intervention in the form of an acute request for a home visit.

7.1.3 Project activity and social care

Approximately 30% required some form of social work intervention, confirming the need for a productive relationship with the social work system. Probably, the most significant challenge at the beginning of this new way of working was overcoming the inherent barriers between the primary health care team and our social work colleagues (2).

We originally incorporated two fully qualified social workers in the MDT structure, one for vulnerable children and families and one for adult services. The very strict eligibility criteria that they were constrained to work under gave rise to some initial conflict, which was resolved by moving to working with social care workers who were less constrained by strict criteria and more able to respond flexibly and quickly to some of the lower level, but nonetheless crucial, preventative measures, that were being highlighted at multidisciplinary team discussions.

7.1.4 GP recruitment and retention

A feature of the project has been the employment of young, recently qualified GPs to act as locums within each practice. These young GPs have found Govan to be an attractive place to work and, as a result, three have become partners within the health centre, replacing recently retired partners who, incidentally, continued to work well into their 60s and were happy to do so in this very positive environment. Seeing young doctors willing to take up partnerships in Deep End Practices has been a gratifying experience for the whole project team.

7.1.5 Conclusion

It is too early to assess long-term outcomes but consistent with the Inverse Care Law, Govan SHIP has helped to identify a substantial group of patients with complex needs, which were not being satisfactorily addressed despite relatively high levels of patient contact. Extended consultation times, increased capacity and improved communication within an extended primary care team have made it possible to re-coordinate and re-invigorate their care.

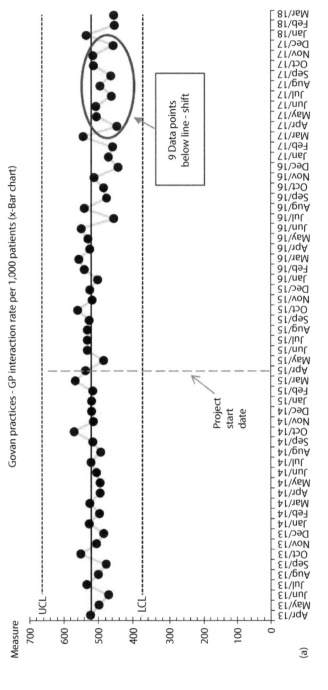

Figure 7.2 GP interactions with patients before and after the start of the (a) SHIP Project in Govan (SHIP) general practices. *(Continued)*

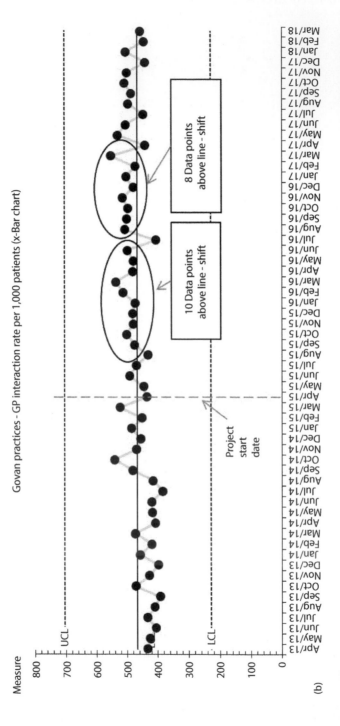

Figure 7.2 (Continued) GP interactions with patients before and after the start of the (b) comparator general practices in Glasgow.

7.1.6 GP use of protected time – 1

AMANDA CONNELLY

In general, GP protected time allowed me to plan clinical reviews of complex patients outside busy surgeries. Time was protected and, therefore, uninterrupted with clear advantages to patients and doctors. In addition to this use of protected time, I wish to highlight one particular clinical case and one clinical development pathway.

The clinical case involved a patient with complex mental health needs. Presentations to health services were chaotic, frequent and often inappropriate. For example, over seven years, this patient presented to A&E on 600 occasions. Contact with primary care took place almost daily. Management was challenging and involved multiple agencies with minimal interagency contact.

Protected time allowed for a difficult but successful negotiation with the patient resulting in an agreed pre-arranged weekly contact of 20 minutes with one GP. A&E attendances reduced from 90 in the year before GP allocated time was introduced to 28 in the year following its introduction.

Regular interagency meetings were arranged and attended by the patient, the GP involved, plus colleagues from psychiatry, social work, criminal justice and A&E Consultant staff. A care plan was agreed across all agencies. Implementation has improved patient care and the management of chaotic unplanned presentations.

The clinical development pathway involved A&E attendances by patients from the four GP practices involved in SHIP. We reviewed inappropriate patient presentations at our local A&E department. It was felt that patients would be better served by having a planned appointment with the practice, thereby avoiding a long wait at A&E followed by redirection back to Primary Care.

A dialogue started between primary care, A&E consultants and the hospital management team. An audit reviewed all A&E attendances over a four-week period. At the end of the four weeks, any attendances thought to be inappropriate were forwarded to the A&E consultant. The consultant reviewed the cases and agreed they could have been safely managed in primary care without any requirement for hospital investigation.

The audit demonstrated that the extra number of patients a practice would need to see per week was only one or two patients. If this was scaled up, the impact and saving on A&E attendances would be significant.

A process of redirecting patients from A&E to primary care was agreed between the four practices involved in SHIP. The redirection policy was agreed to be safe and efficient but could not be implemented at the hospital as it was not possible for hospital staff to run a separate process system for patients from four practices. To be implemented, this approach would require a city-wide policy.

These two examples were only possible because of direct funding for the SHIP Project.

In the first example, a local issue was identified. However, only with protected time, could it be appropriately addressed. The resulting outcome had a positive impact on the patient, the practice, secondary care services and the criminal justice system.

The second example demonstrates the positive development of closer working with our secondary care colleagues. In an overstretched health service, these relationships are crucial for future health care planning.

7.1.7 GP use of protected time – 2

BRIAN MILMORE

Having protected time through Govan SHIP has allowed me to give vulnerable and complex patients the time that we both need to understand and address their problems. Being able to see patients in a busy surgery and openly admit that I cannot deal with everything they present in a ten-minute appointment has been liberating. Being able to offer the patient an extended appointment on a planned basis has allowed me (and often the patient) to prepare better for this encounter and to make it more productive.

I have also been able to contribute to child protection conferences, case conferences for vulnerable adults and assessment of patients cared for under the Mental Health Act in a way, which was not compatible with regimented surgery times and busy day-to-day practice. I hope these contributions facilitate better continuity for patients and they have certainly improved my job satisfaction.

Protected time has also allowed me to develop IT tools to facilitate better ways of working: from better recording of interactions with patients on our clinical systems, to interrogating these systems in more detail than we have had time or resources to do previously. I have had the time to refine these tools, models and searches and then share them with colleagues and further refine them based on feedback. I have learned new IT skills from colleagues within health and social care, contributed my clinical knowledge and experience to how they develop systems moving forward, and hopefully I have helped to create systems that are meaningful for the GPs who then get presented with this information and, more importantly, for the patients who could benefit from any planned interventions based on it.

7.1.8 GP use of protected time – 3

JOHN MONTGOMERY

The Govan SHIP Project began as an idea generated in response to the Scottish Government's proposals to integrate Health and Social Care. As one of the main drivers of the proposal and being willing to take on responsibility for the project's development, my appointment as clinical lead by the participating practices was quickly approved.

The post did not attract any specific additional remuneration either personally or to my practice, but the project provided each GP principal with one session per week of protected time, and leadership activity was incorporated into this. My partners could see benefits to the practice if the project was successful and all have taken leadership roles for some of the work streams associated with the project.

Being seen to be taking part personally in this new way of working as well as continuing my part in other practice responsibilities – clinical work, training, practice administration, and so on – was essential in persuading my partners and the other GPs in the health centre to adopt these quite radical changes to their working life.

Obtaining funding from the government was essential for beginning the project. I had been the elected chair of the South Glasgow GP committee for several years. This body was separate from the Glasgow Local Medical Committee (LMC) and concerned itself purely with health policy decisions in South Glasgow, an area covering 250,000 patients. Having the backing of this committee for the project together, crucially, with the support of senior health service management, social work and academic colleagues allowed us to present a powerful and ultimately successful case to the government.

Positive outcomes rarely result from the actions of a single individual, no matter their leadership qualities, and SHIP is no exception. Our achievements include:

- Achieving additional resources for Deep End practices to attempt to address the Inverse Care Law at a time of financial austerity
- Improving morale amongst experienced principals and enthusing young GPs to take up partnerships within the health centre against the national trend
- Building constructive relationships with a wide variety of health, social and third-sector colleagues and creating a template for extension to other practices regardless of the populations they serve
- Having time to address the unmet need (e.g. poorly coordinated care) in selected patients with improved outcomes

Obstacles have included the need to apply every year for ongoing funding and in doing so having to deal with a succession of new civil servants, albeit with success to date. Longer term funding will be required to achieve the project's full potential.

A Govan SHIP general practice won the RCGP Scotland Practice Team of the Year Award in 2017. The rules of the competition did not permit a collective submission, but the award was considered an accolade for all of the Govan SHIP practices (http://www.sspc.ac.uk/reports/).

7.2 THE DEEP END GP PIONEER SCHEME

PETRA SAMBALE

The scheme involves five participating practices:

- Each general practice has additional clinical capacity (about 10% extra) via a salaried GP fellow
- Each GP fellow works six clinical sessions per week in one of the practices. Three sessions are additional, helping to redress the Inverse Care Law, while three allow protected time for host GPs to engage in practice development

- One of the protected sessions is for a GP lead in each practice
- Practice GP leads and GP fellows meet every six to eight weeks as a group to share experience, views and plans
- Learning is shared among participating practices via an online Trello platform and more widely via engagement with local GP clusters
- Regular day release sessions are attended by GP fellows, with educational content and outcomes posted on Deep End website (See Section 16.6)

I was appointed as a GP coordinator after submitting a formal application and following an informal discussion with the other lead GPs and grant holders. A major part of my role is to coordinate group meetings.

Within practices, there have been many quality improvement activities based on reviews of practice systems and changes appropriate to each practice.

The regular meetings have allowed us to get to know one another, to appreciate the differences in organisational structures within each practice, to build mutual respect and to share learning.

A common concern is to prepare for challenges ahead, e.g. when the GP Pioneer Scheme ends in each practice. General practice is changing with many GPs developing portfolio careers. The Pioneer Scheme provides a breathing space for careful planning to try to ensure that we are fit for the future. GPs and GP Pioneer Fellows both benefit from this opportunity for intergenerational learning and peer support.

We have begun to integrate Practice Managers into the project to give them the opportunity to learn from and share ideas with each other. It is important that GPs avoid spending too much time on tasks that can be carried out by others.

The Scheme has helped to retain and stabilise GPs. Established GPs have repeatedly remarked on how invigorated they feel through working collaboratively with the other participating GPs and with the GP Pioneer Fellows. The established GPs provide positive role models for the GP Pioneer Fellows and have increased their engagement through teaching, including sessions with medical students, which is important if we have to attract new recruits to general practice.

Limitations of the scheme include the lack of administrative support and the lack of funding for external evaluation.

GP leadership is easier in bottom-up projects, as this approach resonates with practices. It is important to understand that although practices work differently, they can learn from each other. However, it is paramount that there is an investment in the time required to build up relationships, define common aims, share experience and develop trust.

GPs are used to observing and adapting their practices to the fast-changing world of medicine. There needs to be an awareness, however, that working in leadership roles within the wider NHS involves a slower pace of learning and change.

The GP Pioneer Scheme is demonstrating that initiatives such as this are paramount for recruitment, retention, quality improvement and for starting the journey of collaboration. A longer time frame is essential, however, ideally five years, if established ways of working need to be overcome following a period of recovery from burnout.

7.2.1 GP use of protected time – 4

JOHN GOLDIE

In the twilight of my career as a GP, our practice successfully applied to host a Deep End Pioneer Fellow. As the lead GP, I was responsible for fostering a supportive, reflective and creative environment where the partners and the Fellow were encouraged to develop initiatives that would enhance the effectiveness of our practice and improve patient care.

Partners appreciated having the time and space afforded by the scheme to reflect on how this could be achieved. We decided to concentrate on developing projects involving one or more GPs and chose projects in clinical areas, service development and health promotion. Some involved reflecting on our appointment and repeat prescribing systems. Others looked at cervical and breast screening arrangements. We audited our management of osteoporosis and non-alcoholic fatty liver disease. We also used the time to tackle diabetic clinic defaulters and frequent attendees at the practice.

Seventy-five patients who had 18 or more items on repeat prescription were reviewed, and individual items were checked for both compliance and appropriateness. 74% of our target group of diabetic clinic defaulters have been reviewed. 41 patients on long-term bisphosphonate treatment, due or overdue a repeat DEXA scan, have been referred for a scan. Four patients had their medication appropriately stopped. GPs have had time to attend social work case conferences that they would not have otherwise had the opportunity to attend.

Having the time and space to reflect, plan, implement and evaluate change has been productive, educational and cathartic. We have shared our experiences and learning with the wider practice team. Team members value the increased variety in their day-to-day work that protected time offers.

I have been energised by the experience and by the enthusiasm and commitment of my partners and the GP Fellow. As a GP nearing retirement, it has motivated me to continue to retirement age. I recommend protected reflective time for all GPs. It would help recruitment and retention issues and improve the quality of patient care.

7.2.2 GP use of protected time – 5

DEBORAH MORRISON

Having protected time during the transition from salaried GP to GP partner has been of immeasurable benefit. It is clear to me that I would have been unlikely to have increased my GP sessions, or committed to becoming a GP partner without this time. This is an important point as I spent the first six years post CCT doing anything but a regular GP job. I was overwhelmed by my registrar year and could not see myself working primarily as a GP. After six years, I realised that I needed to give 'proper' GP another go and decide once and for all whether I could work in frontline primary care.

The practice I joined was transitioning from being a majority full-time to a majority part-time GP practice. Systems that had worked well in the past were no longer fit for purpose, and the consequences were felt particularly by the part-time GPs, who were relatively newly qualified or had taken recent career breaks. Having dedicated time to think through the main issues, be in a position to explore the options, and finally get new systems up and running has been so satisfying. That is not a word I would have used previously to describe my experience of working as a GP.

Importantly, with the protected time, there has been autonomy for the GPs to use these sessions as they see fit. For me, it is about improving systems to improve patient care and reduce practice workload. Other GPs have focussed more on direct patient care projects. Overall, it removes that sense of frustration and powerlessness that feeds into high-stress levels and burnout. From a recruitment point of view, the small reduction in patient contact pays for itself and more.

I can now see how a future in general practice might look for me if protected time is continued. I want to stay in general practice and even envisage increasing my sessions. Previously, I had to choose between using my time in the evenings or weekends to work on practice improvement (sacrificing rest and family time) or 'firefighting' and doing what is needed to get through the day (sacrificing the sense of satisfaction and autonomy that goes along with undertaking practice improvement activities). For now, I do not have to choose.

7.2.3 GP use of protected time – 6

DOUGLAS RIGG

As a full-time GP, the concept of protected time is appealing but daunting. The risk is in trying to achieve too much and inadvertently increasing workload. We set up a practice project board and individual objectives to ensure they meet SMART criteria (Specific, Measurable, Achievable, Relevant, Time-bound).

We had several broad themes including complex case management, quality improvement work at both practitioner and practice level, improving well-being in practice, recruitment and retention and academic work.

Complex case management included extended consultations to allow for more effective management planning, especially anticipatory care. An example is a GP visiting newly registered care home patients to assess medical and social needs. Capacity assessment, legal status, anticipatory care planning, identification and liaising with next of kin, legal guardian or power of attorney and sharing this information via an eKIS platform are all completed. Other examples include input to MDTs or child protection case conferences.

Quality improvement work focuses on clinical and management activities at patient and practice levels, for example, the development of practice guidelines for palliative care and new cancer procedures such as meetings to review referrals for suspected cancer and ensure that all new cancer patients are referred for holistic assessment.

Increasing all GP appointments to 15 minutes has led to an improvement in doctor well-being scores. This has only been possible with the additional clinical input, which has also allowed doctors to move away from their desks to have lunch or get out for a short walk during the day. The impact of this should not be underestimated for retention of GPs. We were also able to host a refugee doctor on clinical attachment to help recruitment to primary care.

I have been able to conduct some practice and cluster level research, which will be used to complete a research project for a Master in Primary Care degree. This led to my engagement in research at the university both as a GP collaborator and as a research participant.

In summary, the Deep End pioneer scheme has allowed me to develop as a clinician, academic and leader and allowed the practice to develop a more effective and holistic and anticipatory approach to care, instead of the previous 'firefighting'. Practice team morale has improved, and we are enjoying the challenges of general practice at the Deep End.

REFERENCES

7.1 The Govan SHIP Project

1. Mercer SW, Fitzpatrick B, Guthrie B, Fenwick E, Grieve E, Lawson K, Boyer N et al. The Care Plus study – A whole system intervention to improve quality of life of primary care patients with multimorbidity in areas of high socioeconomic deprivation: Cluster randomised controlled trial. *BMC Medicine* 2016;14:88.
2. Harris FM, McGregor J, Maxwell M, Mercer S. A qualitative evaluation of the Govan SHIP Project: A social and health integration partnership project. 2017. Downloadable at: http://www.sspc.ac.uk/reports/.

8

Link workers in general practice

An army of people with job titles including link workers, navigators, connectors and organisers has recently been recruited with the general remit of making better use of community resources for health.

This section is based on the experience of link workers working in general practices and making use of practices' contacts with patients and knowledge of their problems. Key components of this approach, which distinguish it from the development of similar roles elsewhere in the community, are the following:

- Embedding the link workers as part of the practice team
- An unconditional approach to patients' problems
- The ability to work one-to-one with patients

A link worker is much more than a signpost to community resources, therefore, and is best considered as an addition to the generalist function in primary care.

The principal features of the Glasgow Link Worker Programme are described below. Experience of working with link workers is then described by Mark Kelvin, the Programme Director; Dr Maria Duffy, whose practice hosted a link worker and Dr Peter Cawston, the GP lead for the Programme.

8.1 BEST ARRANGEMENTS FOR LINK WORKERS

The following commentary is based on the Records of Learning from the Scottish Government-funded Link Worker Programme and captures the essential features of the Link Worker role.

8.1.1 Community link practitioners

- Are employed and managed by a Third Sector Organisation, with a clear governance structure. There is an equal partnership between management and clinical leadership
- Undergo a robust selection process that involves clinicians and GP practices themselves: all current CLPs have a community development background
- Are employed in a senior position (Band 5 KSF Framework) so as to be able to operate as a 'pragmatic socially engaged generalist practitioner'
- Are integrated into the primary care team by a careful process of induction, training, trust building and relationship development
- Work within a clear contractual framework (service level agreement, honorary contract)
- Have NO exclusion criteria-'if it's their problem it's our problem'
- Belong to two teams: the GP practice team and the link workers team
- Go beyond social prescribing or signposting through working with individuals directly to find solutions and overcome barriers as well as providing whatever support may necessary
- Work with individuals to address several issues, either concurrently or over a period of time. To do this effectively, they must possess a range of skills and experience and be able to exercise a high degree of autonomy and professional judgment
- Work alongside people in an open, collaborative non-judgemental manner. This requires personal qualities of warmth, empathy and strong positive communication skills to establish the necessary conditions to address often complex issues
- Contribute to medical records via GP information systems
- Have long appointment durations and scope for being flexible in their approach. This is also crucial in optimising the likelihood of meaningful engagement with individuals and getting to the root of often highly complex and emotional issues
- Meet together every week for peer-to-peer learning and information and knowledge exchange as well as support. This is important for link workers in problem-solving on many fronts
- Meet regularly with their practice team and attend multidisciplinary meetings, practice meetings, practice events
- Play an active role in the development of the whole practice capacity to support patients and undertake social prescribing and signposting
- Build relationships with community resources, gathering and managing intelligence on these
- Are able to provide feedback on local services with a view to service improvement and to develop new responses to unmet need

8.1.2 Key considerations

- GP practices require support to adapt to the new role as this is quite destabilising in the early stages
- Recording and data management requirements, while necessary and useful, can place a significant burden on link worker's capacity
- Each link journey and interaction can vary widely, not least in intensity. Many link interactions are characterised by deeply emotional subject matter, for example, bereavement or trauma
- The 'peeling the onion' phenomena is typical of link journeys in that many underlying issues often come to the fore at various stages in the journey. The senior autonomous role of the link practitioner is essential in ensuring that problems do not bounce back to the generalist practitioner because they are too complex (for example, patients expressing suicidal feelings)
- The resilience of the people whom link practitioners work with is an important motivational factor in what is a busy, emotional and sometimes isolated role

8.1.3 Community-linked practices

- Become oriented towards health and well-being, beginning with the team itself
- Develop the capacity to share learning and for continuous practice development
- Develop their awareness of the barriers and exclusions that patients face daily (especially in our practice systems)
- Develop the ability to process, store and access local intelligence about systems, resources and services for our patients

A Link Practitioner in a GP practice that is not working towards becoming more community-linked is likely to have significantly less impact on patients' well-being and on mitigating the impact of health inequalities.

8.2 EXPERIENCE AS A PROGRAMME DIRECTOR

MARK KELVIN

Third-sector organisations often offer hyper-local, specialised services and support. They are well placed to meet the needs of local populations, but their funding structures can lead to a number of issues. Services are often funded to support people who are experiencing a specific issue, or who are within a particular age range or live in a specified postcode area. Reporting requirements mean that referral pathways vary and can be complex, and the short-term nature of funding means that service accessibility can be unpredictable and inconsistent.

General practice, in contrast, takes all comers. If it's the patient's problem then it's the practice's problem. GP practices have no complicated access criteria, and GPs can support patients from cradle to grave.

Despite their differences, third sector resources and GP practices have one key factor in common. Both offer flexible, reactive, person-centred and relationship-based support, leading to authentic relationships of trust whereby deeper issues are shared, addressed and sometimes resolved. Relationships start face-to-face but quickly progress to working side-by-side.

It was in this context that the Health and Social Care Alliance (Scotland) (The Alliance) and GPs at the Deep End Partnership Link Worker Programme was developed.

It is important to recognise that Link Workers have existed in many guises across Scotland for some time. In the third sector, such roles were often developed in response to the needs of a particular organisation's beneficiaries. For example, the Scottish Consortium for Learning Disability developed Local Area Coordinators to support disabled people, and Alzheimer Scotland developed Post Diagnostic Support Workers to work with people newly diagnosed with dementia. The nature of these roles means that they do not naturally align with the generality of general practice and so cannot easily benefit the practice population.

GPs cannot be expected to remember, nor trust, a plethora of services, referral pathways, access criteria etc. Moreover, with welfare reform and other austerity measures increasingly impacting on primary care presentations, there is a need to support people who may not otherwise be able to access a specialist link worker.

The role of Community Link Practitioner (or CLP – the considered job title given to Deep End GP Link Workers) has been specifically co-designed by GPs at the Deep End and the Alliance to be an effective 'link worker' who is fully embedded as part of the GP team. Co-design has been a critical aspect of the programme.

Community Link Practitioners have three main functions. First, they work with anybody who wants to see them. There are no exclusion criteria. The CLP-Patient relationship lasts for as long as appropriate. Some Link Worker services have a set number of appointments or sessions more akin to acute care than primary care. The CLP aims to develop a meaningful relationship of trust with patients and aims to help them identify any barriers that they are facing to living well. First encounters can last an hour while subsequent appointments vary in length. Given their position as an integral part of the GP team, they often inherit the trust held between GPs and patients and nurture it further. This can lead to issues, different from those given on referral, being disclosed, sometimes for the first time. The CLP will then share the onward journey to access appropriate services that can support the patient to address these issues. For some people, this may be simple 'signposting' or information provision.

Where CLPs benefit the practice population most is in working with people who have not had the opportunity to develop self-determining capacities such as health competence, relatedness and autonomy. People without these skills are less likely to access services by themselves. CLPs can help to augment patients' skills in order to ensure access and use of support and services.

For this to happen, GPs and the practice team must trust the CLP and have confidence in his or her ability to receive referrals, conduct one-to-one encounters and support the patient safely.

Second, CLPs also work with the practice team to work towards seven practice capacities:

- Improving GP team well-being
- Developing shared learning activity
- Increasing awareness of the social and personal context of illness
- Gathering and managing intelligence about local services
- Developing confident signposting behaviours
- Developing networks
- Overcoming local practice problems that could prevent this activity

Trusting the CLP to support this improvement journey is critical. Without wider team support, the CLP can become an add-on service that develops a waiting list and creates another bottleneck in the system.

Third, CLPs have a community development role. They reach out of the hub of general practice into the community and develop relationships across the spokes in order to complete the wheel. These personal relationships between professionals are a powerful tool in enabling the wider primary care team to feel confident in signposting patients to local services.

If Link Workers simply support patients to navigate a fragmented system, the system itself will remain fragmented. By taking a strengths-based approach and enabling the entire practice team and the wider community to support patients to access the right place for them, at the right time, whilst simultaneously offering more personalised support to those who benefit from it, then more parts of the system are navigated more efficiently. It may not fix the system, but it's a co-produced intervention that increases the efficiency of the existing system and supports patients that benefit from it the most and so, it's a start.

8.3 EXPERIENCE AS A HOST PRACTICE

MARIA DUFFY

As GPs, we learn a lot from our patients over many years, listening, making sense of, trying to find solutions or a way forward. We teach our trainees to have a wider understanding of the human condition and that the standard medical models have their place but are reductionist and inadequate in many cases. The Link Approach has given us the tools to address this. We have a trusted colleague (the Community Link Practitioner) to help us explore these areas and enable GPs and our patients to address some of the difficulties they encounter. The readiness of patients and colleagues to embrace this broad social prescribing model is impressive.

My first tentative forays into a referral to the link practitioner with a 'I know this is thinking a bit laterally but …' were met by patients largely with open, willing interest. It felt almost like they already understood but were willing to stick with the medical model (supplemented by my best but rudimentary efforts at social prescribing) as a means of healing, perhaps because that was all that was on offer.

The practice now has effective contact with many organisations, a walking group (and a spin-off patient-initiated and run Arts and Craft Group), weekly visits from community groups and a few visits by us going out to meet community groups in their bases. We have also considered team well-being and introduced a morning coffee break, added extra reception hours, hold walking meetings if possible to reduce sitting time, set aside small packets of time for meetings (rather than trying to add them on while eating lunch and doing house calls between surgeries), an electric bike available for house calls and all four GPs attended the annual UK RCGP conference in Liverpool – 96 years of medicine between us and we had never once been to any RCGP meetings.

I read statistics about the life expectancy of my patients, particularly the young men, and feel we are failing them, the easy to ignore, the homeless, those with severe mental health problems, or drug misuse. I know this project is part of the solution but for some it came too late.

The young man consults, homeless, sofa-surfing, drinking heavily, workless, anxious, looking for something to calm him down. He is agitated, politely insistent that he would feel better with a 'benzo'. His life is, by his own admission, out of control. I have seen him many times before, offered the standard services but I know he will not attend because there is no stability, no effective advocacy.

However, we now have a very capable link practitioner and more in hope than expectation I introduce him. He puts his time and humanity and wit into assisting the young man. The system seems too burdensome to overcome, with barriers at seemingly every turn. The Link Practitioner accompanies him to try to secure stable housing, to keep his benefits, to stop the negative trajectory of his life.

We have a few wins and he knows we are on his side, not just denying him the 'benzos' but actively trying to provide more useful therapeutic interventions. The link practitioner feels outraged at times by the reception they receive while trying to negotiate the systems. There are no exclusions from the Link service, no time limitations. We start to hope.

When the policeman calls with news of his death, I feel profoundly sad and step out of my room to compose myself. I phone his mother. The Link Project had enabled us to be truly empathic, to walk alongside him, to confront the systems he faced, to work through the problems. He died. I believe he died knowing we were advocating for him, not just paying lip service, not just walking on the other side.

8.4 EXPERIENCE AS A GP LEAD

PETER CAWSTON

The programme had seven participating practices across Glasgow City. My role as the GP lead, funded for two sessions per week, had the following elements:

- Leading on the recruitment of practices and link workers and the building of relationships
- Working in partnership with the Health and Social Care Alliance, who hosted the programme and employed the link workers
- Being supported by close working relationships with the programme director, management team and administrative support
- In partnership with colleagues, developing the programme from a general idea to both a theoretical framework and a practical methodology
- Providing enthusiasm, vision and practical support and advice
- Supporting the academic team in developing an evaluation
- Interfacing with the programme executive board, politicians, the media, the Scottish Government, NHS bodies, third-sector organisations and GP practices
- Contributing extensively to academic and documentary papers. Presented the programme at academic, NHs and third-sector conferences

From my point of view, the GP leadership role has been primarily one of influence rather than power. The GP who works in an area of poverty has both profound personal knowledge of the intimate details of peoples' lives and a large-scale perspective through being the head of a team providing services to a deprived population. When this is combined with a grasp of political and theoretical issues, a vision of what the potential of general practice could be, and the ability to express this clearly, the influence can be considerable. A GP does not 'fit' within the established hierarchies of the NHS and can, therefore, unsettle and surprise. I would summarise the GP leadership role as being to provide inspiration and vision grounded in reality and experience. These are a potent combination.

A GP leader can usually only hope to persuade. In the final analysis, those who hold the levers of power are swayed by many different influences. GP leaders need to be prepared to be patient, to take a very long view and to accept disappointment. This is not a failure, but a reality. Willingness to listen and accept the wisdom of others, non-attachment to the outcomes of projects, a sense of perspective, humility and humour are all helpful qualities, although I have certainly not always lived up to this. The most important lesson I would like to pass on to myself from my experiences would be always to deal with others with kindness, no matter how disagreeable the circumstances.

Being given the opportunity to have a GP leadership role is nevertheless profoundly rewarding and life enhancing, and I am very grateful that I have had the opportunity to experience this.

9

Community practice

What good is sitting alone in your room?
Come hear the music play
Life is a cabaret old chum
Come to the cabaret

Sung by Liza Minelli in *Cabaret*
Lyrics by Fred Ebb

This section describes five examples of capacity building within, with and around general practices in communities in Scotland, Ireland, Australia, the United States and Belgium. The practices serve similarly hard-pressed populations in widely different health systems.

Peter Cawston describes measures to improve the well-being, morale and performance of the practice team in Drumchapel, Glasgow – sometimes called 'putting on your own oxygen mask first'. Tom O'Dowd describes starting and building up a Dublin general practice from scratch. Tracey Johnson and Suzanne Williams in Brisbane describe new ways of working with specialist colleagues, including mental health. Andrea Fox and Ken Thompson describe a more fundamental integration of physical and mental health services in Pittsburgh, which we in the United Kingdom can only envy. Finally, Jan De Maeseneer, walking the walk as well as talking the talk, describes a professional lifetime of community engagement and social advocacy in Ghent, Belgium.

9.1 DRUMCHAPEL, SCOTLAND

PETER CAWSTON

There came a moment in our story as a practice team when our sense of who we were and where we were going felt as if it was coming apart in a stormy sea. We felt battered by expectations we couldn't meet, weighed down by needs we should meet, blown about by targets, sinking under rising levels of risk and all the time working more frantically.

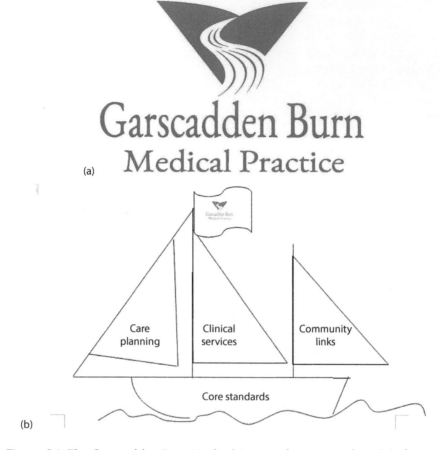

Figure 9.1 The Garscadden Burn Medical Practice logo (a), and model of practice development (b).

As we set out to try and find a way through, it was to this metaphor of a sinking ship that we turned. We could hope that the efforts of politicians and campaigners might deliver calmer seas one day, but in the meantime, we needed to avoid sinking and, if possible, to move forward. So, we literally came up with a boat-based model for our practice development (Figure 9.1).

9.1.1 Let's not sink: Core standards

By all measures, we were performing well. However, a performance is just that – it tells little of what is going on inside. More than a decade of achieving high-performance targets had left us with a weight of neglected basic housekeeping and near chaos in any area not covered by a target. Then, at a very low moment, our practice manager resigned. This possible disaster proved to be a key turning point. For the next three months, we made our focus entirely on long-neglected areas. Sixty black bin bags of sometimes decades old accumulated detritus became symbolic of a complete overhaul in basic housekeeping practices: data storage and management, filing systems, practice policies and much more.

At times of emergency, it is instinctual to neglect routine procedures to face acute challenges, but this response does not work well when crisis is chronic. Housekeeping becomes even more necessary in a hostile environment, like pumping out water taken on board from heavy waves to allow the team to ride the next wave more lightly.

Core standards are about people more than paperwork. An even more damaging instinct is to defer self-care in the face of pressure. The human trait of self-sacrificial response to emergencies is nowhere more admirable than in health care, but when a state of emergency is endemic, self-sacrifice is harmful. Even before our three months of physical clean-up, we had begun to make practical steps towards developing our personal and team housekeeping. The most important of these was taking the decision to close our doors for one afternoon every month.

These monthly 'protected learning time' afternoons have arguably become the single most important activity we now undertake to try and assure our resilience and development as a practice team. It is not always easy amidst the tide of external pressure, but our success in protecting this space allows us every month to 'check in' with the whole practice team, catch up with one another's lives, take care of professional development needs and talk about where we are going.

One outcome of these afternoons was a recognition of the need for protected lunchtimes, with doors closed for an hour, and following this, a decision to introduce a weekly lunchtime yoga class for all the practice team, which is still going strong three years later. A practice well-being policy followed, including buying fruit for the staff room, encouraging physical activity, holding mindfulness classes, and enjoying regular practice meals and celebrations. Most importantly, our development as a practice team started and ended with the recognition that caring for our single greatest asset – us – is our highest priority.

Self-sacrifice is written into most narratives about stressed and overworked GPs. We have needed to keep coming back to this self-care philosophy. The decision to take up yoga and mindfulness has not only supported our physical and emotional health but has also helped to introduce an ethical counterbalance to these cultural pressures. One result has been to open up a dialogue with ourselves about who we are as a practice team, and what kind of GP practice we believe our patients need. This began with a conversation held one afternoon at a protected learning time, asking: 'What kind of future do we want to create?'

9.1.2 Let's move forward: Compassionate services, care planning and community links

It was a revelation in this conversation to discover how far short our day-to-day work fell from the aspirations that we held. Who had created the reality we were working in? Would it be possible to at least imagine a different future? It seemed to us that our work should be primarily one of the caring relationships and not just a series of tasks. The majority of people registered with us face existential threats far greater than we do, living in a socioeconomically deprived peripheral housing estate in Glasgow at a time of national austerity. Many are hindered from fulfilling their own individual exceptional potential in life opportunities and in lifespan. For them, the importance of a practice team lies neither in heroics nor in statistics but in seeing faces they know and having people they trust. It felt strange to talk about compassion and values in the context of practice development. However, finding out what makes us 'tick' as a practice was a great leap forward and has shaped many of our decisions and plans since then.

This internalisation of the locus of control led us to question what high-quality health care means. Collecting and recording of data had become an end in itself, with the purpose out of sight. People with economically impaired life expectancy need a well-organised practice which can deliver good medicine, but this needs to be brought about by good care planning, in which all the team from administrators to senior clinicians feel empowered to do the right thing, not by trying to achieve artificial targets. This will never succeed if patients are treated as passive objects in an impersonal health care delivery machine. 'Care' happens in a symbiotic web between the GP practice team, the local community and third sector, other NHS and statutory services, informal and formal carers and, most importantly, individuals themselves. Practice development has to move beyond internal relationships and systems within the practice team to address this long-neglected, damaged and dysfunctional web of links and relationships.

One consequence of this changed focus has been the development of practice patient groups – not consumer focus groups but patients being supported to find answers to health problems for which we could not offer them a solution. One of these groups identified loneliness as their common health issue and developed into a community befriending group. The other, started by a practice nurse frustrated with the disempowerment, anxiety, cultural norms and poverty that prevent people taking up her advice, has become a peer support holistic lifestyle change group. Both offer small examples of a shifting dynamic in the mutual interdependence between a GP practice and a patient community.

9.1.3 Let's release our exceptional potential

The people who make up our practice team have been our greatest asset. We have found a practice manager with excellent people skills. We have GP partners who have strong values and a willingness to make changes and take risks. We have members of staff who care about people and have been willing to go outside their comfort zone and take on new challenges. Most of this potential was already there. Our practice inherited a long history of multidisciplinary meetings and a culture of caring for individuals. These are not rare to find in general practice. What has changed for us has been discovering that this potential can be released to allow us to begin to develop our own vision of what we could be.

We have had other factors on our side: I have had academic training, which helped me to contribute leadership, analytical and practical skills; the GP partners have used personal connections to help us access expertise and advice; we have been part of the Deep End GP network, providing inspiration and empowerment; through this we were able to become the lead practice in the Link Worker Programme, providing us with new resources, such as a Link Worker, and the opportunity to share our development with other like-minded practices. We have also taken substantial risks. We have invested in additional administrative and clinical capacity, offset in part by accessing new sources of revenue such as short-term grants and providing new services, but also paid for in reduced earnings for the GP partners. When offered the opportunity to leave the national, target-based GP contract and sign a simpler local contract we took this leap, much against the advice of our local medical committee.

Some of these factors have now become part of the landscape of general practice: there are new academic health inequalities fellowships, GP clusters, small networks of GP practices (such as the Pioneer Scheme), link worker posts being created nationally, and a new Scottish GP contract which has abolished target-based remuneration scheme and has promised to invest in additional capacity within general practice.

We are not a unique practice although our story is, of course, an individual one. In 2016, we were awarded the RCGP Scotland Practice Team Award in recognition, we believe, that our experience might resonate with other GP practices in Scotland. We have not reached a safe haven where all is well. This journey continues to be tentative and imperfect, in the face of huge structural problems, such as the Inverse Care Law, which continue to threaten us existentially. Amongst all the contingencies, setbacks and disappointments; however, we now feel that we can work together as a practice team to shape a future of our own, in which we will perhaps one day fulfil this exceptional potential.

> A poor life this, if full of care
> We have no time to stand and stare
>
> **W. H. Davies**

9.2 DUBLIN, IRELAND

TOM O'DOWD

Fifty years after the fight for Irish independence, the population of the Irish State was at its lowest. Immigration had depleted the small towns and parishes with the flight to the cities. The beneficiaries of Irish immigrants were cities in the

United Kingdom, the United States, but also Dublin, which like most capital cities steadily increased in size despite its own poverty.

The increase in population in Dublin led to disastrous planning decisions in the 1970s whose consequences are still evident today. The small rural village of Tallaght in south-west Dublin had 2,500 people which increased to 70,000 over a 15 year period. It was a combination of private and council housing developments with hardly any infrastructure.

In the early 1980s, young single-handed general practitioners began to open up shop in corner houses around housing estates in Tallaght to cater for the health needs of lower-middle-class patients who paid fees for medical care. The location of a practice was left up to a market economy with fee-paying patients getting preference over those covered by the State. In an attempt to improve medical care to socioeconomically deprived patients, the Irish State reformed its general practitioner contract in the 1970s so that patients could choose a doctor. This was cold comfort to patients in under-doctored areas such as Tallaght.

In the 1980s, a Trinity College Dublin health needs assessment in Tallaght found that health needs took third place behind security and jobs. Security was bedevilled by the Irish love of horses which roamed the area in a semi-feral state causing injury to local people. The Trinity study led to the establishment of a horse project which taught local young men to look after horses with some eventually becoming employed as jockeys and stud hands.

A more recent community needs study in the 1990s showed that health had now become a major concern, especially general practitioner services. GPs were, as now, very popular with patients but there were not enough of them. One of the districts in Talllaght, Jobstown, had a population of approximately 16,000 but no local health or GP services. Despite its name, it was an area of high unemployment and blighted by the emerging heroin epidemic in Dublin. Following the publication of the Trinity College health needs assessment which, importantly, went down a political route, a large health centre was built quickly by the Health Service Executive with the support of a charity, the Mercer's Foundation. The health centre became a focus for health services such as nursing, speech and language therapy, psychology, psychiatry, dentistry and physiotherapy. However, because of the fee structure of Irish general practice, GPs were not expected to work there and indeed were unwilling to do so. As a local general practitioner and academic, I was approached to provide GP services on a part-time basis for a year to see if it was possible and viable. Seventeen years later, I continue to be the, now senior, general practitioner in the practice, along with three younger colleagues, a nurse and administrative staff.

From the start, the practice was established on modern lines with an appointment system, and trained reception, management and nursing staff. We established a tolerant but firm approach towards bad behaviour as outbursts upset waiting patients much more than we expected. Every patient is personally called into the consulting room by the clinician which creates a presence of the doctor or nurse in the place and a sense of availability.

A consultation with a patient who lives in a deprived area, with high levels of local crime, attendant anxiety and significant family, educational and health problems is often difficult. It is impossible to provide a holistic consultation within the constraints of modern general practice. We try to focus on the clinical content and provide other services such as social work and psychology for more specialised input. However, the default rates with such services are high. The intensity of clinical work and the associated exhaustion have not led to close working relationships with psychology and social work. There seems to be an oil and water mix between GPs and primary care staff in terms of patient demand, ways of working and indeed methods of remuneration. As GPs we don't have the inclination for meetings and have a fear of being given responsibility for complex families that is beyond our resources. The other professions try and leverage the GP/patient relationship which can seem to us like passing the buck. Despite having access to more primary care facilities than many GPs and despite wanting to practice in a more rounded manner, we have become more traditional than we planned at the outset. Patients have a view of health care which in our case has proven to be conservative and to which we have perhaps too easily responded. We have recently put social prescribing and practice-based pharmacy in place which is being taken up with GP encouragement.

At the centre of the practice is confidentiality. Working in an area with drugs misuse inevitably leads to crime, which has a ripple effect within and between families. Our health centre has become a place of refuge where people say things that in other circumstances would be of importance to investigating police. It does mean advising patients to be careful about what they say to us and agreeing with them what we enter into their files.

Our programmes have been of value to our patients. Our methadone programme has become integrated into daily practice and has allowed patients to get on with often productive lives. Childhood vaccination rates are at 92% and we have universal folic acid adherence in early pregnancy. We have an active contraceptive approach and have not had an early teen pregnancy in the last ten years. In response to our high suicide rates, we have established a men's health clinic that is well supported by the community. This charity-supported clinic is GP-led with a psychologist and sees a large number of traumatised young men who are all too eager to choose a pharmacological approach to their problems.

At a local level, health issues often involve local politicians, some of whom became patients. They have been supportive but largely adopt the mantra 'if it ain't broke, don't fix it'. Their main focus is our local hospital with its variable performance, long waiting lists and overcrowded emergency department. We got criticism from politicians prior to setting up a local out of hours co-op but after being established the issue is now off their agenda.

The guidance of occasional health needs assessments and an ear to the ground has led to the development of a service that has been extended to another centre in the last two years. None of us works full time in the practice, which has helped us cope with the demands of the clinical and psychosocial needs of the area. Having wider academic, clinical and business roles has given us a combined skill set and networks that benefit patients and the practice. These wider roles have prolonged our clinical usefulness and grounded our contributions to general practice at local and national levels.

9.3 BRISBANE, AUSTRALIA

TRACEY JOHNSON AND SUZANNE WILLIAMS

Inala Primary Care (IPC) is a charitable general practice in the western suburbs of Brisbane, the capital of Queensland. The 'western suburbs' are synonymous in Australia with disadvantaged communities as they are furthest from the coast. Many, like Inala, are becoming infamous for social dysfunction and rising racial tension. Forty-nine percent of IPC's 4300 patients live in the bottom 10% of household incomes and more than two-thirds live on pensions or receive benefits.

From a general practice perspective, that means they hold a 'concession card', providing evidence they have limited capacity to pay out-of-pocket expenses. For this reason, IPC sends daily invoices to the Office of Medicare in the Department of Health to claim for services rendered – a business model called 'bulk billing'. Practices in more affluent areas submit 'mixed bills' meaning they charge most of their patients around double the Medicare scheduled fee. A claim is then sent to Medicare with the patient receiving the Medicare rebate within five days and bearing the remainder of the cost personally. Medicare rebates have been frozen in Australia for the last five years.

General practice is wedged between revenue pressure and increasing patient complexity. As a fragmented collection of over 7,000 individual businesses, general practice in Australia is poorly positioned to lobby for change. IPC is a canary in the coal mine as patients are 60% more likely to have diabetes (1) and up to three times more likely to smoke (2). So, despite Australia having a universal health care system rated as one of the top four in the world (3), patients in catchments like Inala experience the Inverse Care Law every day.

Bulk billing providers typically schedule eight or more patients per hour per doctor and employ few nurses. This is because the Medicare schedule rewards shorter consultations. This is obvious when the various item numbers are graphed against the time triggers associated with each and revenue per minute is calculated (Figure 9.2). Patients of greater complexity attend IPC because we never schedule more than four patients per hour and make extensive use of the higher value chronic disease item Medicare numbers which support management planning. Our charitable status offsets some taxation expenses and our mission and models of care attract doctors prepared to work for less in order to deliver more. Despite affording patients more time, as occurs in mixed billing practices, we struggle for sustainability.

In a volume-based funding system, there is little incentive to add value. However, access to public endocrine departments for patients with uncontrolled diabetes is becoming a national challenge. A decade ago, patients referred by IPC waited over nine months. This led to the practice partnering with the hospital to generate what is now termed a 'beacon model of care'.

The hospital provides a Diabetes Educator, who screens and supports patients throughout the week. On Tuesday mornings, three upskilled GPs working under endocrinologist supervision see 24–36 patients depending upon the new to

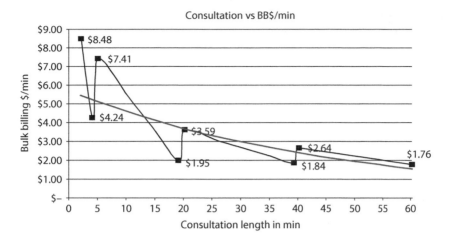

Figure 9.2 Medicare reimbursement by consultation length.

review ratio. Onsite podiatry triages and commences care. Patients commencing insulin are supported by the Diabetes Educator with results viewed by GPs the following week. Patients reaching their targets are discharged for ongoing care by their referring GP.

Studies show that IPC's beacon model of care, taking referrals from 23 postcodes, costs around half the cost of the equivalent hospital outpatient model (4). It also reduces avoidable admissions to hospital by half, with no show rates being one-third of outpatient attendance. The model has been replicated in two sites reducing average wait time for an endocrine referral to less than one month. Rotation of one of the three GPs each year ensures surrounding practices have the opportunity to upskill and collaborate.

Based on this result, IPC implemented a similar model for renal disease using an upskilled practice nurse and three GPs supervised by a Nephrologist. The Keeping Kidneys model was independently evaluated by Deloitte Access Economics and having been recommended for rollout, has recently been included in the statewide renal plan.

Lessons from these models include:

- Focus on diseases with the demand to sustain a revolving cohort of around 200 patients to maximise the productivity of the visiting physician and divert hospital funding
- Medicare will not fund the time to create and coordinate such services. Hospitals need to contribute funding
- Engage specialists with a vision to improve access and the patient experience
- Enlist GPs willing to upskill, work systematically within a multidisciplinary team and adapt to refine the model
- Create an evaluation strategy at inception so that a business case can be established

- Employ nurses with superior communication and organisational skills, as the models of care need to be managed between the clinics, GPs and attending specialists
- Patient education and support can be provided by nurses and alter disease trajectories
- Hospital physicians gradually come to appreciate GPs as clinical generalists, so that GP's breadth of skills and patient relationships can be harnessed

Obesity is a challenge in the Western world, especially in western suburbs. IPC has developed an obesity pathway, which involves overweight patients attending their GP for a management plan. Patients attend four visits per year with their GP and obtain education and support through matched visits with practice nurses. Patients are referred for Medicare-funded visits to a dietician and an exercise physiologist. A nurse-led, six-session group preventative health program is also offered. The systematised development of patient knowledge and group identification aims to support the adoption of new behaviours.

Stemming the tide of chronic disease is especially important in a practice already supporting one of the most complex patient groups in the country. Twenty-eight percent of patients visit the practice more than 12 times per year, meaning that 1300 patients need to receive intensive support.

GPs feared routine screening was being overlooked whilst managing the polypharmacy and social complexity of patients. This led to the practice of offering patients a Preventative Health Check which ensures that immunisations, screening and periodic investigations for conditions outside their main chronic disease are attended to. The service is nurse-led and has reduced the number of unplanned extended visits to GPs. Patients look forward to this opportunity and often require short follow-on visits with their GP to receive referrals for screening, imaging or pathology.

For the last nine years, IPC has had a resident mental health nurse caring for complex patients. Support for between 45 and 70 patients with chronic and complex mental health issues is offered in a step-up, step-down fashion. Two psychologists deliver six sessions each week utilising Medicare funding to deliver 10 visits annually to patients eligible for a Mental Health Care Plan. Embedded mental health providers are fundamental to our care given the coalescence of chronic disease and mental health issues.

We are planning the collection of Adverse Childhood Experience (ACE) scores (Section 11.3.3) in our practice. This will improve identification of children at risk of long-term chronic conditions, build support for high ACE parents and target care to the most vulnerable patients. We are also embedding a community legal service to prevent the cascade into worse mental health and disengagement from care which results from life stress. This will diffuse some of the complex consultations our GPs face with patients in desperate housing, domestic violence, and drug- and debt-related circumstances.

Through the REMAIN HOME Project, the practice has a part-time non-dispensing pharmacist, with the role of reconciling medications after hospital discharge, providing patient education and support to GPs in managing complex medication schedules and advising authorities of adverse drug events.

Australia is engaged in a staged rollout of tiered bundled payments for patients with chronic conditions called the Health Care Home Program. With around half of our 4,300 patients eligible, we anticipate redesign of the practice layout, increased multidisciplinary teamwork and expansion into digital health once the program arrives. The clinical redesign, project management, research, governance, collaboration and communication skills all need enhancement to support our team move into population management.

IPC has evolved an array of dashboards over the last five years. Managed through a Clinical Governance Committee and GP theme leaders, our embrace of evidence-based medicine created work teams inclined towards evidence-based management. Our approach has been positively received, highlighting that benchmarks and data will be embraced if practitioners consider them relevant in practice.

Critical to supporting our work has been time for our senior leaders to undertake study tours, collaborate across the health sector, improve their management skills and thinking process. Increasing funding constraints are limiting these necessary activities at the very time that primary care is becoming more dynamic. To get beyond the silos, to improve productivity and to increase patient and clinician satisfaction we need to invest now.

9.4 PITTSBURGH, PENNSYLVANIA

ANDREA FOX AND KENNETH THOMPSON

During 'the war on poverty' in the mid-1960s, the US Congress created a number of programs to enable poor people, disabled people and people over 65 to access health care. Some are very well known. Medicare is a federal program that pays for health care for older and disabled people. Medicaid is a combined state and federally financed program that pays for health care for people living on incomes below the poverty line (increased in some states to 137% of poverty by the Affordable Care Act). Neither of these programs, however, actually provides clinical services and many people in need are not eligible for them.

To partially fill this gap in access to treatment, Congress authorised funding to create a network of community mental health centers (CMHCs) and then community health centers, now called Federally Qualified Health Centers (FQHCs), to provide community-based mental health care and primary medical care, respectively. Funded in different ways by a complex mix of federal, state and philanthropic dollars, CMHCs and FQHCs generally serve people with high needs. The FQHCs receive additional federal funds requiring them to see people without insurance. There is no requirement that CMHCs and FQHCs in the same community connect with each other in any way.

Over time, a number of things became increasingly apparent. First and foremost, people with psychiatric challenges routinely came to FQHCs for medical care. This number increased as more people with psychiatric challenges left hospitals and lived in the community and as more psychiatric conditions such as depression, developmental disabilities, dementia, PTSD, substance use disorders and even psychotic disorders were recognised by primary care medical practitioners. At the same time, as psychiatric medications entered into their armamentariums, it became easier for primary medical practitioners to provide limited forms of psychiatric treatment. Many did so. Of course, these openings encouraged further growth in the number of people with psychiatric challenges attending FQHCs. A similar phenomenon occurred in the CMHCs, where people with medical problems were seen on a daily basis. However, unlike the FQHCs which developed some response to the presence of psychiatric challenges in their patients, relatively few mental health centers did the reverse and developed mechanisms to provide medical care. Very few FQHCs or CMHCs sought out partnerships with their opposite number.

In recent years, as these issues of epidemiology and practice have become more clear, it has been finally recognised that health care for people could not be rationally divided at the neck, as it were, and that the 'silo-ed' approach of separating 'physical health services' from 'behavioral health services' impaired the ability of either service to care for people effectively and efficiently. Integration of behavioral health care with primary medical care has become the watchword across the United States, fueling significant efforts to combine both systems of care. Numerous initiatives are underway to find ways to provide the whole person, whole life primary health care, combining behavioral and physical health care that is coordinated and connected to family and community resources. What follows is a description of an effort to fuse psychiatric and medical care into true primary health care in an FQHC in Pittsburgh.

The Squirrel Hill Health Center (SHHC) is one of almost 1,400 Federally Qualified Healthcare Centers operating at approximately 10,000 service sites across the United States. Each FQHC is required to provide preventive and primary health services to anyone who walks in their doors, in addition to making linkages to necessary services outside the FQHC. They can provide psychiatric services if they so choose. In fulfillment of these and other quality and quantity requirements, they receive a lump sum payment from the federal government on a yearly basis plus cost-based reimbursement through Medicaid.

The SHHC was approved for funding 12 years ago with a mission to care for all who came but with special attention to socially excluded people with challenges of access to care due to language, cultural barriers or limited mobility or capability, such as homebound older adults. The SHHC's start coincided with a marked increase in both immigrants and refugees resettling in Pittsburgh, which was still recovering from the demise of the steel industry.

As might be expected from our mission, immigrants, refugees, uninsured Pittsburghers and older adults make up the core of our patient population. Given their social marginality, many have comorbid medical disorders, psychiatric challenges and complex social circumstances. In response to this profile of patients, we have had to develop a 'health home' that provides an array of services onsite that many either cannot afford outside the SHHC walls or encounter too many obstacles to assemble themselves. As a result, we now see ourselves as providing coordinated whole life primary medical and dental care, including women's health services, fused with behavioral health care, which includes medically assisted treatment for addictions.

To our way of thinking, both 'physical' and 'behavioral' health care have primary and specialty components. This may be more thought out in medicine than psychiatry, which has focused on its specialty status. Much of our immediate challenge has been to figure out how much psychiatry and what kind of psychiatry fits best in a primary health care setting that serves populations with very significant psychiatric challenges in addition to medical ones.

In our setting, we have decided that the need for psychiatric expertise and capacity is more than that can be expected from generalist physicians who are focused on treating physical illnesses, even with additional support, such as a behavioral health liaison worker. We have also decided that the simple co-location of services is not sufficient and that the interface of medical, psychiatric and social issues in our patients is far too interdigitated to carve out entirely separate medical and psychiatric realms. We have opted instead to do our best to 'fuse' services – to connect the head and the body – in how we think and act as much as possible. As a result, we share workspace and medical records and meet formally and informally throughout our work. When possible and necessary, we see patients together.

Over time, given the growth of our patient population (25,000 visits a year by 7,000 patients, 65% of whom speak a primary language other than English), we have added more medical and psychiatric capacity. At present, we have three primary care medical physicians, four nurse practitioners and three physician assistants with associated support staff. We have one half-time psychiatrist, a full-time psychiatric nurse practitioner, three therapists (all social workers), a behavioural health coordinator and four or five part-time peer support workers. With this array of resources, we are able to conjointly manage a wide range of medical and psychiatric disorders.

Much has been written about the clash of cultures when combining behavioral health care and primary medical services. While we found that the pace of work varied and adjustments had to be made in scheduling on both sides, we found that our guiding principles of care – focused on recovery-oriented care and the activated patient in the context of family and community – were entirely compatible. It has become clear to us that fusing our work allows us to really find the person in person-centered care. The person's life story is a vital sign.

Despite ongoing resource constraints and volatility, we are hopeful about the future and our ability to continue improving our services to people in need who seek community oriented whole person 'fused' primary health care. Perhaps with a little luck, this approach will be able to truly take root in Pittsburgh and the United States.

9.5 GHENT, BELGIUM

JAN DE MAESENEER

When my wife and I graduated in 1978, we started a practice in Ledeberg, which in those days was one of the most deprived areas of the city of Ghent in Belgium. As students, we had been investigating new ways for making sense of the profession of medicine, and the obvious choice we made was to become general practitioners and work in a primary health care team, with the aim of building an inter-professional community health center. Later, in 1978 we read in the Alma-Ata Declaration (1) that what we were trying to do was exactly what the Declaration was describing: engaging with local communities, addressing the upstream causes of ill health, investing in the empowerment of citizens and patients and integration of care.

A first challenge was to develop in-home care by teams of different professionals, working together to address the bio-psycho-social needs of vulnerable people. In our daily consultations as general practitioners, nurses and social workers, we were confronted with the impact of poverty on patients' lives. So, in 1986, we put poverty on the agenda of the local authorities and brought together all care providers, but also representatives of schools, police, social institutions, informal caregivers and ethnic-cultural minority groups, in a platform that met every three months in order to exchange information and formulate a 'Community Diagnosis'.

The challenges we had to address included the poor physical condition of the youngsters, as observed in daily consultations and documented in a survey to be due to lack of physical activity. Bringing all the stakeholders together led to a clear diagnosis that there were almost no green spaces in the densely populated neighborhood. The prescription was not vitamins or physiotherapy, but the construction of playgrounds and the organization of activities during school holidays. The assessment of this intervention brought three conclusions: the police reported less 'street-criminality' during the holidays; the physical condition of the youngsters improved and, interestingly, different ethnic communities met around the playground activities, contributing to better intercultural understanding.

Other challenges were traffic safety, addressing epidemics of lice and scabies and, later, tackling the poor dental condition of the youngsters. When family physicians examined children's throats and mouths, they often observed the disastrous state of their teeth. A cross-sectional study of 30-month-old toddlers indicated that 18% had early childhood caries (2). Children whose parents had lower education, lower-ranking jobs, lower incomes and were living in more deprived neighborhoods had a significantly higher risk of early childhood caries. Children whose mother had an East European nationality had even higher prevalence rates. This study was one of the decisive arguments to integrate accessible dental care in the Community Health Center in 2006. Moreover, the Flemish government decided to integrate dental screening at 30 months in the official program of 'Well-baby and Child clinics'.

All these interventions illustrated the strength of the Community-Oriented Primary Care approach (COPC) whereby, starting from data registered in the daily consultations of physicians, nurses and social workers, a 'Community Diagnosis' is made and together with the local population, interventions are planned and their impact monitored (3). COPC integrates individual and population-based care, blending clinical skills of practitioners with epidemiology, preventive medicine and health promotion, minimising the separation between public health and individual health care.

Already early in the development of the Community Health Center, it became clear that fee-for-service was not the appropriate way to fund the integrated approach to primary health care which we were developing. In 1982, therefore, we started to negotiate a capitation system that in 2013 was transformed into a system called 'Integrated Needs-Based Capitation'. Based on the data recorded by the insurers, every year a 'picture' is made of the population on the list of the center, and 42 variables are used to indicate the 'average care-needs' of this population. On this basis, an integrated capitation is provided for general practice, nurse and physiotherapy. Other professionals such as health promoters, social workers, tabacologists, nutritionists and community health workers are paid via different financing streams.

Advocacy has always been an important task of the health center. Giving a voice to the voiceless became increasingly important, as the last 20 years saw an increase from 25 nationalities in the community to 107. So, every consultation is a journey around the world and it is important that the many signals captured in consultations and revealing social welfare and health system problems are translated into local policy, first at the level of the community, and if that is not sufficient, in the City Health Council. Direct interaction with local authorities and even with regional and federal authorities, is needed in order to tackle increasing social disparities.

In the last two decades, there has been an important increase in multimorbidity. We discovered that disease-specific guidelines are not able to address the complexity of people with multimorbidity. Therefore, the practice engaged in a search for the implementation of 'Goal-Oriented Care', starting from the life-goals of the patients, and trying to discover, together with the patients, what interventions are appropriate in order to achieve those goals (4). Goal-Oriented Care requires fundamental changes, not only in care processes but also in the way we structure our information, as the goals of the patient become an essential component linked to episodes of care (5).

Recent years have seen more and more integration with social care in addressing issues of health and welfare. Very often, the general practitioner and the social worker become the central axis in the process of this integration. Moreover, with the development of Primary Care Zones in Flanders, primary care providers become more and more accountable for a geographically defined population (±100,000 people). This accountability requires more integration between primary care and public health services.

But there is more. Nowadays, in times when people are increasingly confronted with violence, with fragmentation, with opposition between 'WE' and 'THEY', the response of general practice and primary care will have to be based on solidarity, on respect for diversity, on building bridges instead of walls, on establishing 'connectedness' (6). General practitioners and primary care teams can make a difference by building trust, strengthening coordination, contributing to continuity, demonstrating flexibility, being responsive to a diversity of needs and demands, engaging in advocacy and demonstration of leadership in societal change processes.

The simple fact is that a citizen in Ledeberg knows, when he is in trouble, that he can go, either to the Community Health Center, or to the Social Welfare Center, and that he/she will be treated respectfully by skilled, empathetic professional people, giving him/her the feeling that he/she is 'part of a society' and that 'everybody counts'. This contribution to social cohesion that we have been able to make in the past 40 years in the community of Ledeberg is a continuous inspiration and source of energy: 'We can together imagine a better future, we can make it happen'.

REFERENCES

9.3 Brisbane, Australia

1. Australia's Health Tracker by Socio-Economic Status: A brief report card on preventable chronic diseases, conditions and their risk factors, Tracking Progress for a healthier Australia by 2025. Australian Health Policy Collaboration, 2017. p. 5.
2. *WORNA: Whole of Region Needs Assessment.* Eight Mile Plains, Australia: Brisbane South Primary Health Network, 2017.
3. Mirror, Mirror on the Wall, 2014 Update: How the US Health Care System Compares Internationally, Exhibit ES-1 Overall Ranking, 2014. http://www.commonwealthfund.org/publications/fund-reports/2014/jun/mirror-mirror (accessed 3 March 2018).
4. Zhang, Donald, Baxter, Ware, Burridge, Russell and Jackson, Impact of an integrated model of care on potentially preventable hospitalisations for people with Type 2 diabetes mellitus. *Diabet Med* 2015;32:872–880. doi:10.1111/dme.12705.

9.5 Ghent, Belgium

1. World Health Organization/UNICEF. Primary Health Care: Report of the International Conference on Primary Health Care. Alma-Ata, USSR 6-12 September 1978. Health for All Series, No 1. Geneva, Switzerland: WHO, 1978. http://www.who.int/publications/almaata_declaration_en.pdf.
2. Willems S, Vanobbergen J, Martens L, De Maeseneer J. The independent impact of household- and neighborhood-based social determinants on early childhood caries. A cross-sectional study of inner city children. *Fam Community Health* 2005;28(2):168–175.
3. Rhyne R, Bogue R, Kukulka G, Fulmer H (Eds.). *Community-Oriented Primary Care: Health Care for the 21st Century.* Washington, DC: American Public Health Association, 1998.
4. De Maeseneer J, Boeckxstaens P. James Mackenzie Lecture 2011: Multimorbidity, Goal-Oriented Care and Equity. *Br J Gen Pract* 2012;62:522.
5. Nagykaldi ZJ, Tange H, De Maeseneer J. Moving from problem-oriented to goal-directed health records. *Ann Fam Med* 2018;16:155–159. doi:10.1370/afm.2180.
6. De Maeseneer J. *Family Medicine and Primary Care at the Crossroads of Societal Change.* Leuven, Belgium: LannooCampus Publishers, 2017.

10

Learning health systems

The task of health care is to produce better health and social value. When interventions have been proved effective in individual patients, the challenge is to deliver these interventions for every patient who can benefit. The key to such care is information, evaluating performance and coverage rates and feeding this information back to practitioners. Learning health systems are not only a technological challenge, they also require cultural change. In general practice, such change is more likely when general practitioners are involved in setting the agenda and asking the questions. In this section, John Robson, Kambiz Boomla and Sally Hull describe over a decade of work developing a learning health system that, impressively, includes all general practices in East London.

10.1 LEARNING HEALTH SYSTEMS

JOHN ROBSON, KAMBIZ BOOMLA AND SALLY HULL

The use of near real-time routine data in electronic health records creates new opportunities for clinical intervention as well as administration and research, for example, shared record views, clinical decision support, safety alerts, precision medicine, optimising medicines and reducing delays in care pathways (1,2).

This has been termed as a Learning Health System, which is a clinically orientated system in which information technology and analytic capability are the key elements, combining and enriching data from a variety of sources and turning this knowledge into improved practice (3). However, this is not simply a software 'plug-in', nor does it depend on passive retrospective data collections that have characterised most current 'big data' uses for planning, administration and research, including the Quality and Outcomes Framework (4).

A Learning Health System is contingent upon a dynamic 'virtuous cycle' starting with the clinician–patient interface and dependent upon trusted inter-disciplinary and inter-organisational interaction, alignment and transparency, as well as advanced and secure data systems, data linkage and analytic capacity. This is a complex translational pathway to produce more informed, smarter and more efficient working. Data is turned into knowledge, and this knowledge informs better practice. It brings together big data from multiple sources including GP, hospital and community care with wider linkage to an increasing array of social information such as social services or Local Authority school records and from patients themselves (5) (Figure 10.1).

More recently, additional linkage to biomedical 'omics', personal apps (such as medicine reminders or self-measurement), wearables (such as Fitbits), environmental exposures (for example, air quality) and disease registers, mortality statistics or research cohorts are all in scope. These sources form an increasingly rich data resource, providing clinicians with real-time information to optimise clinical interventions and care for patient benefit, as well as new opportunities for commissioners, research and population health (6).

From the 1980s, primary care electronic health records in the UK NHS have led the way internationally. In hospitals, with the exception of the national imaging PACS system and some local initiatives, digital development had largely stalled since 2002 (7). In contrast, the last decade has seen some providers in the United States, take the next step in digital maturity to develop more integrated clinical hospital and community digital record systems; for example, Geisinger in Pennsylvania, Intermountain in Utah and Partners Healthcare in

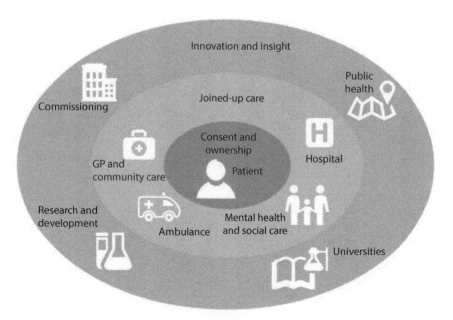

Figure 10.1 Data into knowledge, knowledge into practice; across populations, organisations and disciplines. (From: Greater Manchester Datawell.) *(Continued)*

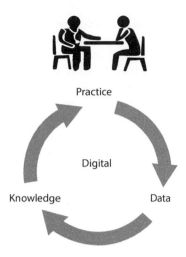

Figure 10.1 (Continued) Data into knowledge, knowledge into practice; across populations, organisations and disciplines.

Massachusetts who have ambitions for extension into wider population-based 'accountable care'.

In the United States, this has stimulated major university, industry and government funding for innovation in learning health systems, including both the technical platform infrastructure for data integration and the analytic/clinical capacity for programming, 'machine learning', natural language processing and other clinically informed data science which generate actionable clinical and organisational intelligence (8,9).

NHS England has been slow to follow, relying on administrative data such as Hospital Episode Statistics, rather than clinical systems, to drive clinical improvement. The imperative to create and utilise interoperable real-time clinical records in the NHS and related services was eloquently summarised in 2016 in the Wachter report (2).

The digitisation of care has been stimulated by opportunity and necessity. The technical and organisational developments associated with the industrialisation of health care provide opportunities while demographic pressures and austerity, with an increasingly aged and multimorbid population in an increasingly resource-constrained health system, generate a necessity for smarter working (10,11). Numbers of patients per GP practice increased by 17% in the decade to 2015. Despite acknowledgment of the key role of primary care in health service systems, the proportion of NHS spending devoted to general practice declined over that period, reducing from 10% in 2004 to 8% in 2015, with some belated increases since but not to previous levels, leading by 2016 to a workload crisis in both primary and hospital care (12–14).

The response in English primary care has been to attempt to work on a larger scale and on a more integrated and smarter basis. Federated general practices are increasingly developing to gain better value and better coordination of services including community and hospital care. Models include federations, networks, alliance, collaborations, companies and consortia (15). Single-handed practices reduced by 50% in 2004–2016, increasing the proportion of practices serving 12,000 or more patients by 20%. Increasing numbers of practices are linked in networks and federations with requirements for cross-organisational appointment systems, patient records and data analysis (12). A recent Nuffield Trust review described the contextual factors driving larger scale collaboration (16). This shift to larger organisations echoes the corporatisation of primary care which took place in the 1980s in the United States (17).

In the context of scaling up general practice, there have been concerns about the geographical footprint of accessible primary care services – keeping GP providers local and within pram-pushing distance – with digitally connected systems including telemedicine and virtual clinics, proposed as more relevant alternatives to centralised bricks and mortar. In 2006, recommendations for primary care in London, including new multi-provider polyclinics serving populations of around 50,000, were considered by many GPs to erode attributes such as access and continuity of care. In response, the Royal College of General Practitioners published recommendations supporting geographically devolved but federated working with a requirement for more integrated data systems (18). Since 2009, the national scope has widened with multiple initiatives testing new models of care with limited evaluation (19,20).

In NHS England, Clinical Commissioning Groups (CCGs), usually coterminous with local authority boroughs, are responsible for hospital, GP and community care, serving populations of about 300,000. In 2013, the public health departments, previously with NHS primary care, were transferred to Local Authorities and most of the IT for planning and commissioning was moved into larger Commissioning Support Units, covering regional populations of around five million.

This reduced the staffing of the new Clinical Commissioning Groups by about a third and greatly reduced their capacity to develop their own organisational or clinical intelligence. The loss of public health and IT 'intelligence' led to stagnation in many primary care information services. A few notable localities retained some in-house IT capacity or support, and these often formed the basis for developing new models of care in subsequent vanguard initiatives (19).

The 2014 NHS England Five Year Forward View and subsequent 2017 Next Steps set out new government strategies towards larger administrative units with populations of around two to five million typically covering upwards of seven CCGs, with a movement towards wider integrated accountable care partnerships including local authorities (21). In 2015, a range of new models of integrated care was funded by NHS England for which digitisation was an integral element; Tower Hamlets in East London was one of these (19).

The political environment in NHS England has become increasingly marketised. To bid for available contracts, GPs in each of the three East London CCGs, like most other areas in England, formed themselves into federated GP organisations with a single contract with their CCG rather than each practice contracting separately (Tower Hamlets Care Group, City & Hackney Confederation and Newham Health Collaborative). In addition, the NHS England Sustainable Transformation Plan had begun by 2017 to create a pan-CCG network to fit the Five Year Forward Plan for larger commissioning organisations typically covering populations of two to three million. In East London, the seven local CCGs were aligned in a new East London Health and Care Partnership with plans to form new alliances with Local Authority services, under the heading of accountable care partnerships (22,23).

By 2016, there were other emerging UK initiatives towards Learning Health Systems aiming to integrate health and social care – for example, the Salford Integrated Record, Greater Manchester Academic Health Science Network and Connected Cities initiatives, seeking to connect health and social services using digital technologies (24–26). The 2016 Wachter review further reinforced the need for digital technologies in the NHS as a fundamental and inter-operable infrastructure supporting pan-organisational care pathways (2). Virtual clinics, Skype consultations and telemedicine have become commonplace in many areas (1). However, inter-operable records continued to elude most of these initiatives. Typically, electronic GP referral letters to hospitals are still printed on arrival and scanned in as attachments to the hospital record.

The Wachter Report pointed out that digitisation is part of a system, not a plug-in, and that

… implementing health IT is one of the most complex adaptive changes in the history of health care, and perhaps of any industry. Adaptive change involves substantial and long-lasting engagement between the leaders implementing the changes and the individuals on the front lines who are tasked with making them work. (2)

10.2 ACHIEVEMENTS IN EAST LONDON

JOHN ROBSON, KAMBIZ BOOMLA AND SALLY HULL

The inner East London boroughs Tower Hamlets, Newham and City and Hackney include GPs in 140 general practices in three Clinical Commissioning Groups (CCGs) (1). They have achieved exceptional success in a number of clinical areas including top ranking in the national Quality and Outcomes Framework (QOF), which is all the more impressive as these CCGs are responsible for a population of 1 million people who are among the most disadvantaged and socially diverse in the United Kingdom.

The population is exceptionally young and mobile, and over half do not have English as a first language. A total of 30% of the population are South Asian and 10% are black African/Caribbean. In these boroughs, 35% of children live in poverty and rates of ill health are among the highest in Western Europe. One in three children are obese at age 11, and 8% of adults have type 2 diabetes. Newham has a higher prevalence of tuberculosis than anywhere else in Western Europe.

Prior to 2008, the GP practices in these three areas often performed in the lowest quintile of national performance. However, over the past decade, GP care in these three CCGs has been among the most improved in England and ranked first, second or third nationally in 25% of the 60 clinical Quality and Outcome Framework indicators in 2016/17 (1–5).

What these three CCGs have in common is support from a university-based Clinical Effectiveness Group (CEG) for the digital maturity of primary care electronic health records and digitally enabled improvement. Although the early success of Tower Hamlets in association with the use of managed practice networks has been well publicised, the success of neighbouring City and Hackney CCG who did not use networks has been equally impressive, pushing Tower Hamlets into second place in the 2016/17 QOF results. Newham CCG also did well without such extensive network support. CEG support is not a software plug-in. It is a system with key elements aimed to change organisational and professional behaviour, aligning capability, action and motivation to achieve 'wise choices'.

10.2.1 Quality improvement: Choosing wisely

The Clinical Effectiveness Group encouraged 'choosing wisely', aiming to support topics which had a robust evidence base, had high impact and value for money, were feasible, often building on existing programmes and had clear performance and evaluation indicators that would show quick wins within three years.

The first programmes in Tower Hamlets were network-supported enhanced services for diabetes and childhood immunisation in 2009 and COPD and cardiovascular diseases in 2010. Similar enhanced services were developed in City and Hackney and Newham from 2010 onwards. Significant improvement in outcomes for these conditions were achieved, including rapid achievement of over 90% coverage and hence community immunity for measles, mumps, and rubella immunization (Figure 10.2), increased use of care plans, and some of the best and fastest improving performance for major long-term conditions in London and England (6).

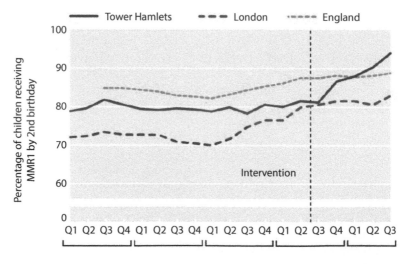

Figure 10.2 MMR immunization, Tower Hamlets CCG, London and England 2006–2010.

10.2.2 Cardiovascular disease

Cardiovascular diseases are the major ameliorable diseases, and medical treatment has the greatest impact on reducing hospital admissions or deaths of any medically feasible intervention. Figure 10.3 shows the proportion of people with diabetes with serum cholesterol below 5 mmol/L from 2005–2016 as recorded in the English QOF. Until around 2008, the three East London CCGs were all below the England average but by 2011 were all well above the average, with the gap continuing to increase. The other local East London CCGs, Havering, Redbridge and Barking and Dagenham shown in 2016, were all below the London and England average in Figure 10.3.

Figure 10.4 shows that Tower Hamlets had the highest capita spending on statins in the United Kingdom with City and Hackney and Newham not far behind, with a widening gap compared to most CCGs from 2014–2016.

In people with CVD or diabetes, we aimed to increase the use of high-intensity atorvastatin when it came off patent in 2016. The three East London CCGs have been among the highest prescribers of atorvastatin in England with continuing improvement. Bradford did even better by taking a decision to transfer all patients to atorvastatin, which shows that even further improvement is achievable (Figure 10.5).

Blood pressure control was another local priority promoted using the same methods to promote alignment of capability, action and motivation. Tower Hamlets and City and Hackney CCGs rank 1st and 2nd out of all 209 CCGs in England for blood pressure control in hypertension, cardiovascular disease and diabetes, and Newham is in the top centile.

Figure 10.6 shows the performance of all CCGs in England by Index of Multiple Deprivation (a measure of socioeconomic status) in the 2015/16 QOF for blood pressure control in people with coronary heart disease, with more

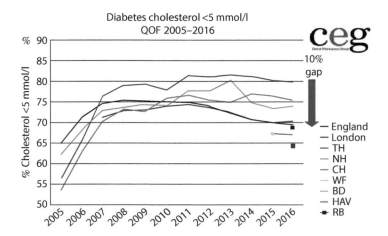

Figure 10.3 Proportion of people with diabetes and serum cholesterol <5 mmol/l. East London CCGs compared to London and England. (Quality and Outcomes Framework 2005–2016.)

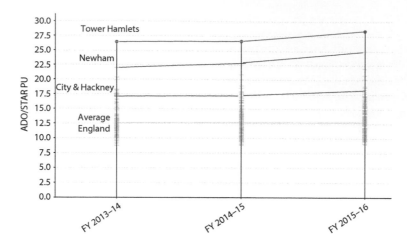

Figure 10.4 Statin prescribing: Average Daily Quantity per standard prescribing unit: All CCGs in England 2015–2016.

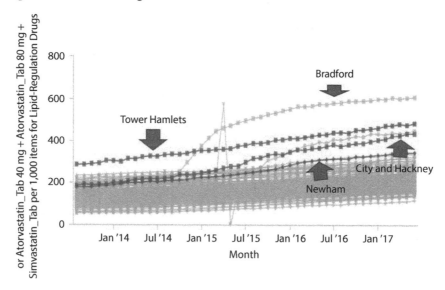

Figure 10.5 Use of atorvastatin 40/80 mg per 1,000 items of all lipid medicines. East London and English CCGs. (From Openprescribing.net.)

affluent areas to the left and more deprived areas to the right. East London CCGs are above the average by 5% and above similarly disadvantaged CCGs by 10%. The average year-on-year increase in the QOF indices is typically 1% per annum so that a 10% gap equates to a 10-year lead by East London CCGs over similarly disadvantaged areas.

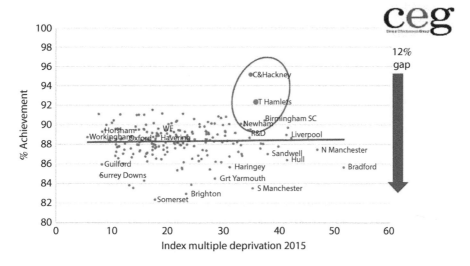

Figure 10.6 Blood pressure control <150/90 in people with coronary heart disease: QOF 2015. All CCGs in England by Index of Material Deprivation. (From Quality and Outcomes Framework and NHS Digital, Leeds, UK.)

10.2.3 Atrial fibrillation

Anticoagulation for atrial fibrillation has been another major local focus for improvement, with the three CCGs having among the best performance in London.

Figure 10.7 is a CEG dashboard for practices in the four CCGs (Waltham Forest was included from 2016) showing improvement in the management of patients with atrial fibrillation. Aspirin monotherapy (now an obsolete therapy) was reduced by more than half in three years – from 25% in 2013 to less than 10% in 2017; and anticoagulation increased by 15% from 63 to 78% as patients were switched from aspirin to anticoagulants.

A programme of pulse regularity checks (opportunistic by manual palpation when checking blood pressure) in people 65 years and older was instituted in all three CCGs, rapidly resulting in a culture change in recording, with 90% receiving a pulse regularity check within five years and an increase of 9% in the atrial fibrillation register size within three years – comprising an additional 790 more patients identified with AF across the three CCGs.

This was achieved by making it easy to record, putting 'pulse regular/irregular' on all data entry templates for long-term conditions, NHS Health Checks and new patient checks and providing on-screen prompts, dashboards and a small financial incentive.

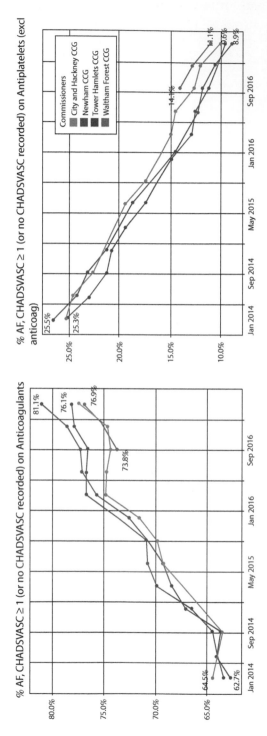

Figure 10.7 Use of anticoagulants and aspirin monotherapy in people with atrial fibrillation CHADSVASC 1 or more in four East London CCGs 2014–2017. (From Clinical Effectiveness Group Dashboard 2017.)

Funnel plots in Figure 10.8a describe performance in Newham CCG who ran this programme, compared to next-door Waltham Forest CCG which did not have a programme. It shows the difference achieved within three years in Newham – no-one was 'left behind' – the culture had changed and the entire distribution improved with reduced variation; pulse checks had become the new normal. Figure 10.8b shows similar data for Tower Hamlets in dashboard

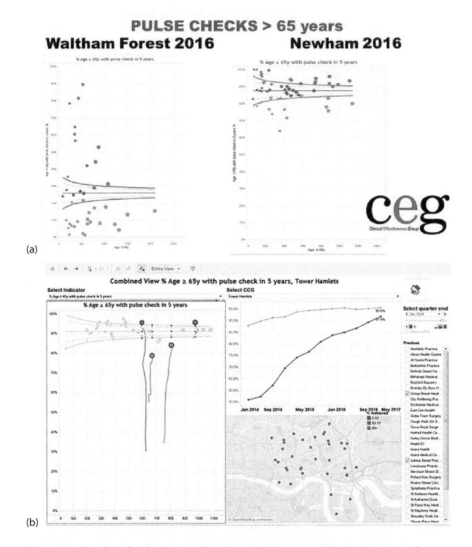

Figure 10.8 Pulse checks in people over 65 years in Waltham Forest and Newham (a), and 'the distance travelled' by individual practices (b). (From Clinical Effectiveness Group QMUL, London, UK.)

format an illustration not only the final achievement but also the 'added value' for practices, illustrating that some had 'travelled' much further than others from 2014–2017.

10.2.4 Reduced inappropriate diagnostic testing

We have also concentrated on reducing unnecessary or obsolete diagnostic testing to cut workload, cost and potential patient harm. This includes reductions in unnecessary liver function tests and blood glucose self-testing.

A 20% reduction in all liver function testing was simply and rapidly achieved by more prudent routine testing for statin monitoring. Routine liver function tests for statin monitoring account for about 40% of all liver function testing, and a full array of six to seven analytes are 'bundled' as 'LFTs' which is the only ordering option. In fact, only a single analyte, alanine transaminase (ALT), is required for statin monitoring, reducing cost and unnecessary testing by a factor of six with further reduction in testing by ending unnecessary routine annual testing. In Tower Hamlets CCG this saved £130,000 within a year, by making ALT an option to order and using the same system of guidelines and digital enablement (7).

The reduction of blood glucose self-monitoring in people with type 2 diabetes not on insulin has been another notable success achieved without any national prioritisation or additional funding in the East London CCGs. Self-testing for type 2 diabetes is, after insulin, the most expensive part of diabetes care. Free machines supplied by the companies are handed out by pharmacies and in diabetes clinics, thus 'locking-in' patients to a lifetime supply of expensive testing strips.

We developed a stakeholder consensus among all local diabetes GP leads, consultants, specialist nurses and prescribing advisors to reduce this use of self-testing where it was not appropriate. A programme supported by guidelines, education, the usual digital prompts and dashboards reduced testing in people with type 2 diabetes not on insulin from 55% to less than 10% in the two intervention CCGs. Newham acted as a natural 'control' as it did not initially take part (Figure 10.9). If replicated nationally this would avoid unnecessary testing in 340,000 people and reduce prescribing costs by £21.8 million per annum (8).

Similar programmes for medicines optimisation have been run to reduce long-acting analogue insulin, inappropriate use of inhaled steroids in COPD and non-steroidal anti-inflammatory drugs.

10.2.5 International comparisons

These results are not only nationally good but are becoming internationally excellent. The results of East London performance in 2015 compared with the USA performance metrics in Healthcare Effectiveness Data and Information Set (HEDIS) for Kaiser Permanente, Southern California, one of the most prestigious of American health care providers, are shown below in Figure 10.10. Results in the selected indicators were at least as good in East

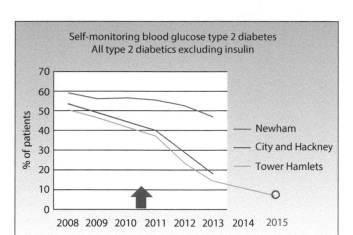

Figure 10.9 Reduction in self-testing of blood glucose in type 2 diabetes not on insulin – City and Hackney and Tower Hamlets with Newham as a non-participating 'control'. (From Wallace, E. et al., *Br. Med. J.*, 352, h6817, 2016; Clinical Effectiveness Group QMUL.)

Kaiser Permanente
S. California.
2015 Top 10% USA

vs East London

	Kaiser	Tower Hamlets	C&Hackney
Diabetes HbA1c <9%	76%	80%	81%
COPD Spirometry	81%	82%	89%
Child imms 2yrs	89%	94%	90%

ceg

Figure 10.10 Kaiser Permanente versus East London CCGs for selected HEDIS and QOF indicators 2015. (From QOF and HEDIS 2015.)

London if not better – and East London covered the entire population, of whom around 20–30% would be excluded in the United States.

10.2.6 Population surveillance and patient safety

CEG has developed trigger tools for declining renal function (Figure 10.11). These are run monthly in practices to identify patients with impaired renal function (eGFR <60 mL/min), who have deteriorated more than 10 mL/min from their previous test. Some of these individuals are already known to the GP but some surprise results have been identified. GPs can refer these patients with

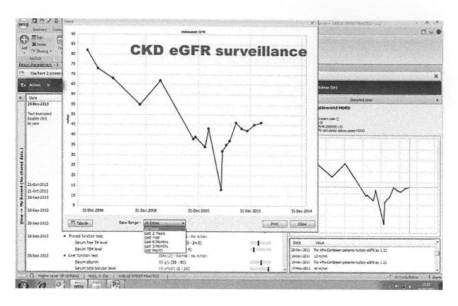

Figure 10.11 Renal surveillance in at-risk patients and the 'virtual' clinic. Screenshot of electronic patient record (EMIS). (From Clinical Effectiveness Group, London, UK.)

concerning renal deterioration into a 'virtual' renal clinic where the consultant renal physicians also use EMIS, can see the whole GP electronic health record including free text and can write a comment. This enables the consultant to write a suggested management plan in the record that the GP can read and act on. Many of these 'virtual' patients are elderly and no longer need to travel further than their GP surgery. Waiting times for the consultant clinical opinion have been reduced from six weeks to less than five days.

10.2.7 The next step

In East London, the existing digital developments are among the most advanced nationally. Owing to the increased capability in primary care, the hospital system has made major advances with 80,000 shared record views every month, with GPs viewing summaries of hospital records and hospital staff viewing summaries of GP records. These shared views are transformative for direct clinical care and the A&E or ward staff can at a click, see the summary of patient record including major past problems and medication. However, although the record is viewed, the data are not integrated – that requires a further step in digital maturity to create a new integrated data service called Discovery.

The Discovery programme provides a technical data platform that integrates all the local health data sources such as GP, community, out of hours and local authority data with hospital records data. This is a real-time system fit for clinical purpose and will drive digital improvement, research and commissioning intelligence in the next decade (Figure 10.12).

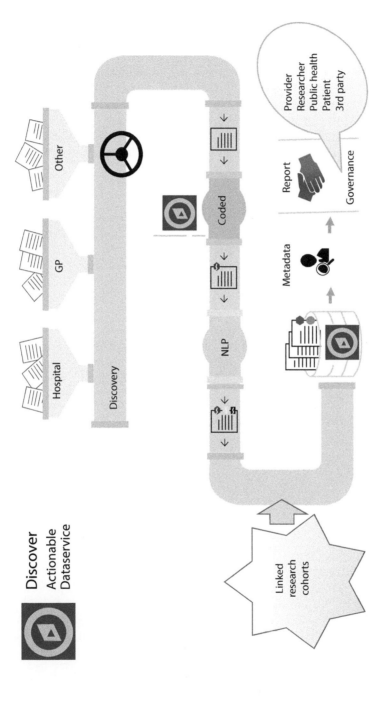

Figure 10.12 A dataservice for integrated clinical care and a learning health system.

10.3 DEVELOPMENT IN EAST LONDON

JOHN ROBSON, KAMBIZ BOOMLA AND SALLY HULL

The success of quality improvement in Tower Hamlets, Newham and City and Hackney and the development of a Learning Health System has been contingent upon several factors including local GP champions, farsighted Clinical Commissioning Group (CCG) administrators and a 'wise choice' of target conditions to ensure early success. A further common factor in all three CCGs has been facilitated support for digital enablement by the Clinical Effectiveness Group (CEG). Together, these factors have formed the components of a learning health system which can actively respond to the needs of both patients and providers.

10.3.1 The clinical effectiveness group (CEG)

Funded by the local CCGs, the Clinical Effectiveness Group (CEG) based in the Centre for Primary Care and Population Health in the local university has been working in East London since 1985 to promote quality improvement using digitally enhanced services. By 2009, almost all local practices used EMIS as a single GP computer system with web-based data extraction, enabling clinical decision-support and real-time reporting of performance, typically monthly or quarterly. Led by three part-time local GP principals, the CEG employed three data analysts and three facilitators, one for each CCG, together with a manager and secretarial support. With CEG support, GPs and practice staff became familiar with and trusted the accuracy, utility and governance around uses of their data.

There have been four key synergistic elements to the success of the improvement programmes.

- **Capability**   Stakeholder 'wise choices' for evidence-based and ameliorable topics yielding quick wins
- **Action**   Facilitated IT support for implementation
- **Motivation**   Reporting and evaluation of peer performance and resourcing achievement
- **Leadership and trust**   Generating ownership, engagement and alignment of initiatives

Building a context for trust and facilitation was essential in permitting the commissioners and providers to take risks on change. Trust enabled CCGs to risk the money and practices to take on the work and risk exposing their performance. 'Quick wins' aligned to existing programmes in immunisation and blood pressure control, led to willingness to develop more complex programmes. Not all programmes were chosen so wisely or succeeded, some falling under the spell of 'top-down' political exigency rather than clinical evidence.

10.3.2 Capability and alignment

Capability included stakeholder engagement, consensus on key performance indicators and organisational alignment of goals across both primary care and the local hospitals. An example of this was the local decision in 2005 to improve the use of statins. At the time, these were prescribed to only 65% of people known to have coronary heart disease or stroke. In a meeting convened with hospital consultants, prescribing advisors, GPs, specialist nurses and CCG and hospital administrative staff, it was agreed that the target should be over 80%.

It was also agreed that this would be achieved using simvastatin, then off-patent and recommended by NICE at lowest acquisition cost, rather than on-patent atorvastatin which cost more than ten times as much. Despite atorvastatin being favoured by many hospital consultants, a consensus was agreed to prescribe generic simvastatin, recognising a minority of individual circumstances and instances in which atorvastatin might be chosen. This avoided bankrupting the local health economy without compromising population health benefits which were rapidly achieved, exceeding the statin target of 80%.

The next task was to formulate a consensus on a set of key performance indicators agreed by the CCG and GPs and set out in an enhanced service including financial incentives on achieving targets. This was summarised in printed and online guidance sent to all practices, with further support in educational clinical meetings (1).

All new enhanced services were developed in this way through local consensus and support via educational activities, including Multidisciplinary Team Meetings (with paid time for hospital consultant attendance) and protected learning time to release primary care staff to attend.

As far as possible new programmes were aligned with existing initiatives such as the national Quality and Outcomes Framework, the local prescribing incentive schemes for GPs and Quality Improvement Programmes in hospital so that GPs were rewarded by achieving both the existing schemes and additionally by achieving the 'stretch' or new targets.

10.3.3 Actionable care – Data entry templates

Standardised data entry templates designed by CEG are used by all practices ensuring both high-quality coding and the agreed items to be recorded. Templates are a major factor in clinical decision support, including coding options, 'hyperlinks' that open documents at a single keystroke (for example, HbA1c values in both old and new mmol/mol values or a guideline/care pathway), structured diagnostic pathways and the ability to generate standard referral letters or care plans. Smart templates are designed for comorbidities; for example, in a patient with diabetes, dementia, COPD and atrial fibrillation a smart template contains all the relevant fields for that patient with those particular conditions, avoiding the need to open multiple templates. Templates may also contain embedded patient leaflets that can be printed and information for clinical staff about referral options as well as 'self-populating' referral letters that include information drawn from the medical record – past history, medication, key measurements or lab results, and so on.

A large range of other 'enhanced services,' whereby practices are incentivised to reach targets for particular conditions, are supported by templates including child and adult immunisation, sexual health, NHS Health Checks, minor surgery and substance misuse. There are also developmental programmes for latent TB testing, rapid HIV testing and domestic violence. Each CCG has slightly different enhanced services but the core of most of them is similar. The template specifications are freely available on the CEG website (2), and the templates are 'open source', authored and maintained by CEG staff with central uploading and national accessibility by any practice using the EMIS electronic health record. Updates to templates can be centrally controlled.

10.3.4 Actionable care – Facilitators

The CEG facilitators are the indispensable spinal cord that connect GP practices to the CCG-designed programmes. Facilitators are often recruited from local practices and are trained in digital support. They are a necessary and key factor in successful implementation, training practice staff in new programmes and providing continuing support. Facilitators provide the detail of coding, templates, and practice organisation including the patient searches and recall schedules required to deliver a coherent programme. They also produce baseline searches showing the variability and average practice performance at a point in time so that targets and finances 'fit' with the CCG budgetary projection for the year. The facilitators make at least two visits a year to each practice (some practices require more visits than others). They also provide telephone support, educational workshops in each CCG and workshops in clusters or networks of practices where these exist.

The CEG also supports a large public health intelligence function which informs local authority needs assessment and planning priorities. Accredited public health staff directly access a CEG database of standard disease and demographic metrics at both ward and practice level. For Commissioners, CEG supports the development of a new service, its evaluation and practice payments and provides continuing support for existing programmes which are annually reviewed and modified over time.

10.3.5 Actionable care – Dashboards and tools

As well as the data entry templates, the CEG has designed software tools to identify eligible people who were, for example, not on statins, using standard searches. Practice computer protocols generated in-consultation 'pop-up' alerts if eligible patients were not on statins and prescribing alerts advised simvastatin as the drug of first choice.

Quarterly dashboards, which showed the performance of all practices in the CCG, were circulated to practices, networks and the CCG, including bar charts, trends and funnel plots (Figure 10.13). In two years, Tower Hamlets CCG had

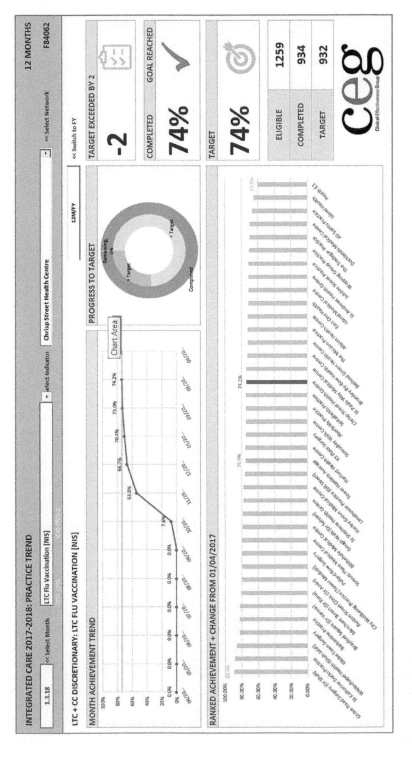

Figure 10.13 Example of a typical dashboard.

attained the 80% target for statins in people with cardiovascular diseases with further subsequent increases by all three CCGs. City and Hackney and Newham achieved similar success using these tools.

An additional software tool was the Active Patient Link tool for atrial fibrillation. This is a search for people with atrial fibrillation undertaken in the practice, the results of which are displayed in a programmed spreadsheet (Excel or Tableau) showing patient details – for example, those on aspirin monotherapy with a high risk of stroke who would benefit from an anticoagulant. Relevant issues such as palliative care, dementia, housebound, comorbidities, bleeding risks and control of blood pressure and statin use are all displayed, allowing rapid triaging of patients for review either by the GP or a visiting pharmacist. Similar tools for heart failure, COPD, hypoglycaemic risk and identification of renal failure were also developed.

10.3.6 Motivation and alignment

Four main elements provided motivation – leadership and consensus between clinicians and managers on the clinical importance of a programme; financial resource via enhanced and similar services; alignment of the programme across and within organisations; and rapid and trusted feedback on performance.

CCG local enhanced services pay additional money to achieve a target above the existing baseline attainment. This system was in place in all three CCGs though only Tower Hamlets used network rather than practice attainment as a basis for payment. Key performance indicators were displayed in quarterly performance dashboards which showed near real-time performance e.g.

- Every practice identified, allowing comparison with each other, using trends, funnel plots and bar charts.
- For an individual practice – 'How am I driving' in that quarter.
- 'How far have I got to go' (e.g. another 50 patients to achieve the higher target of target 91% by 1st April).

GPs have agreed that their dashboards should identify practices for internal peer review within the three CCGs, but they preferred to de-identify publicly available dashboards The dashboards were also used to calculate payments automatically so that practices could send an invoice to the CCG claiming their payment in a way that could be audited, if required, and reduced CCG administration time.

10.3.7 GP practice managed networks and the NHS landscape in England

The delivery of service improvement has differed in some important respects in each of these three CCGs. In 2008/2009, following a relative increase in primary care funding under the Brown Government, Tower Hamlets CCG funded a large investment into eight managed networks, each of four to five GP practices grouped in geographic localities, with the aim of improving care for chronic disease. Each had a network manager and administrative support for enhanced services for diabetes, lung disease, children's immunisation and cardiovascular disease. The practices were typically paid 70% 'up-front' for the service and the remaining 30% if they achieved the agreed target – and the achievement was on the basis of network achievement rather than individual practice achievement. The key interventions included the use of network dashboards which enabled inter-practice scrutiny and interventions for improvement. These were supported by the CEG (funded by the CCGs) to provide IT support for practices enabling rapid cycle review – a key component of a learning health system (3).

There were rapid early successes in these programmes in Tower Hamlets, but over the succeeding decade, these were fully matched by neighbouring City and Hackney CCG which achieved equivalent results without the use of any such networks. Newham CCG also showed substantial improvement, again without major investment in practice networks. Finances in Newham and City and Hackney were kept at practice level and there was no system of network managers as employed in Tower Hamlets. Newham faced the greatest organisational challenges of these three CCGs, including the greatest growth in a highly mobile and ethnically diverse population, served by an older GP workforce often operating from single or two-person practices. Newham has also shown very substantial improvement with performance in the top centile nationally.

10.3.8 What made the difference? Components of improvement

Good local clinical champions and supportive CCG management were undoubtedly important. Tower Hamlets networks made a rapid initial improvement, but Newham and City and Hackney caught up without this support. CEG digital support was the main factor common to all three CCGs and played a central role. Although digital enhancement is a necessary component of the system of improvement, its successful use is contingent on other key behavioural factors such as trust, capability, action, motivation and organisational alignment which together provide the theoretical basis for successful organisational improvement (4–6).

The CCGs and the Clinical Effectiveness Group have a 25-year history of collaborative digital working in these three CCGs – how transferable is this? The CEG is now working in the other four East London CCGs, being careful to 'choose wisely' to ensure some clear early successes on standard programmes such as diabetes and atrial fibrillation. We expect it to take three years to build engagement and trust with the new CCGs and the GPs in the new provider 'federations' in order to achieve a fuller set of competencies across all major clinical conditions. Southwark CCG is building a similar organisation so this is beginning to appear beyond East London and many other CCGs use elements of these methods to promote improvement.

'Choosing Wisely', the title of an American programme reducing low-value care, is a key issue (7). It is easy to get sidetracked into trying to 'boil the ocean' and sort out the political mantra of the moment rather than evidence-based policies. In 2014, the local CCGs were mandated to support 'integrated care' based on an American idea that because 80% of the health care resources were used by 20% of high-risk patients, targeting these high-risk patients would reduce hospital admission (8).

Over the last three decades, there has been little or no evidence to support generic admissions avoidance in high-risk patients. Trials aiming to reduce admission have been universally negative (though patient satisfaction is improved) (9). If there is any effect of generic interventions, it is small and best related to specific treatments for specific conditions such as heart failure, often delivered by highly trained specialist nurses (10). Targeting a relatively small number of people at very high risk of hospital admission with at best a small effect means that the net impact of any such programme will be small.

To have an important effect on events or admissions requires a common condition and an intervention with a large effect – cardiovascular disease fits both these criteria. Optimising CVD prevention has a far greater effect on reducing hospital admission. Medical treatment has been responsible for almost half of the three-fold reduction in CVD mortality in the last three decades (11).

10.3.9 Trust and leadership

The programmes aimed to win the trust of the GPs, who were the data providers, by supporting them to work smarter for greater patient benefit at reduced cost – and at the same time, increase GP income. The neutral university location of the 'honest-broker' function of the CEG helped reduce GP anxieties about performance 'policing' by commissioners and commissioner anxieties about GP 'gaming'. The ability to audit transparently any data extracted reassured practices and provided a means to verify data in relation to payment if this was disputed by the practice.

Trust has been further strengthened by CEG leaders, who worked locally as GP principals, had part-time academic appointments in the university and also held prominent positions as clinical leads in the area. They supported both the CCG to design clinical services and the CEG to deliver these to practices. Clinical leadership influenced the uptake of data-sharing agreements with all GPs, brokering agreements with hospital clinicians about care pathways and prescribing, and getting CCG administrators to risk supporting novel programmes that required additional funding. Effective clinical leadership has also been a major feature in American health care improvement digital initiatives and was highlighted in the Wachter report (12–15).

The university location has also been a major factor in promoting federated data linkage between hospital, GP and local authority data. In all cases, the data controllership has remained with the GPs who remain stakeholders in all data uses. This contrasts with the current situation with the national Hospital Episode Statistic dataset where controllership is transferred from the original hospital controllers to NHS Digital centrally. This creates considerable additional complexity about permissions for third-party data uses. There is much further work to be undertaken, particularly with regard to informing and engaging patients in their access to and uses of their data.

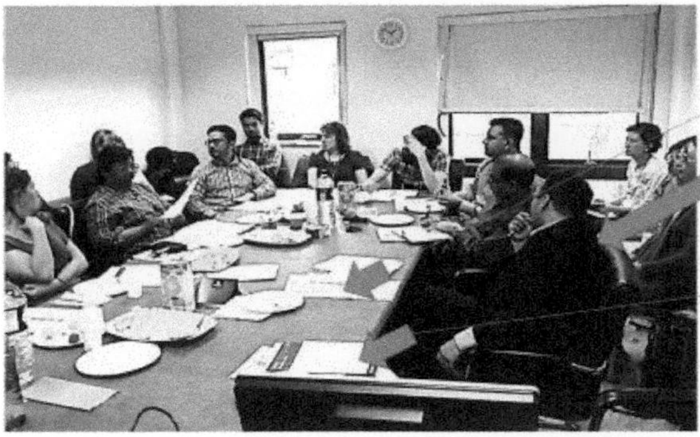

Figure 10.14 A Learning Health System: Discussing diabetes targets in a local MDT.

At the end of the day, the final common pathway involves clinicians and their teams serving individual and population health. Figure 10.14 shows a multidisciplinary team meeting in East London with GPs, nurses, practice managers and a consultant diabetologist looking at new clinical guidance and discussing performance charts of their own performance for HbA1c control and blood pressure. This is what a learning health system looks like – a digitally mature process of organisational change, which enables and informs the discussions that change clinical behaviour.

ACKNOWLEDGEMENT

The Clinical Effectiveness Group is led by John Robson, Sally Hull and Kambiz Boomla and the staff are managed by Keith Prescott. The achievement in East London is entirely down to the vision and trust of the GPs and their staff, the local CCGs and the hospital consultants and administration. This is now extending to include engagement with Local Authorities and a wide range of researchers.

REFERENCES

10.1 Learning health systems

1. Chambers R, Schmid M. Making technology-enabled health care work in general practice. *Br J Gen Pract* 2018;68:108–109.
2. Wachter RM. Making IT work: Harnessing the power of health information technology to improve care in England. Report of the National Advisory Group on Health Information Technology in England: National Advisory Group on Health Information Technology in England, 2016.
3. Friedman C, Rigby M. Conceptualising and creating a global learning health system. *Int J Med Inform* 2013;82:e63–e71.

4. Roland M, Guthrie B. Quality and Outcomes Framework: What have we learnt? *BMJ* 2016;354:i4060.
5. McManus RJ, Mant J, Franssen M, Nickless A, Schwartz C, Hodgkinson J et al. Efficacy of self-monitored blood pressure, with or without telemonitoring, for titration of antihypertensive medication (TASMINH4): An unmasked randomised controlled trial. *Lancet* 2018;391:949–959.
6. Califf RM, Robb MA, Bindman AB, Briggs JP, Collins FS, Conway PH et al. Transforming evidence generation to support health and health care decisions. *N Engl J Med* 2016;375:2395–2400.
7. Knapton S. How the NHS got it so wrong with care.data. *Daily Telegraph*, 2016. https://www.telegraph.co.uk/science/2016/07/07/how-the-nhs-got-it-so-wrong-with-caredata/ (Accessed 26 February 2018).
8. Schilling B. The Federal Government has put billions into promoting electronic health record use: How is it going? Commonwealth Fund, 2011. http://www.commonwealthfund.org/publications/newsletters/quality-matters/2011/june-july-2011/in-focus (Accessed 26 February 2018).
9. Agarwal S, Milch B, Van Kiuken S. The US stimulus program: Taking medical records online. McKinsey Corporation, 2009. https://www.mckinsey.com/industries/healthcare-systems-and-services/our-insights/the-us-stimulus-program-taking-medical-records-online (Accessed 26 February 2018).
10. Pollock AM. *NHS Plc: The Privatisation of Our Health Care*. London, UK: Verso Books, 2005.
11. Hart JT. *The Political Economy of Health Care: A Clinical Perspective*. Bristol, UK: Policy Press, 2006.
12. Health and Social Care Information Centre. General practice trends in UK to 2016, 2017.
13. Iacobucci G. Ministers in 'denial' over NHS crisis. *BMJ* 2016;353:i2507.
14. Roland M, Everington S. Tackling the crisis in general practice. *BMJ* 2016;352:i942.
15. GP Online. Huge surge in GP collaboration to deliver services at scale, 2015. https://www.gponline.com/exclusive-huge-surge-gp-collaboration-deliver-services-scale/article/1374975.
16. Rosen R, Kumpunen S, Curry N, Davies A, Pettigrew L, Kossarova L. Is bigger better, Lessons for large-scale general practice: Nuffield Trust, 2016. https://www.nuffieldtrust.org.uk/files/2017-01/large-scale-general-practice-web-final.pdf.
17. Himmelstein DU, Woolhandler S, Hellander I. *Bleeding the Patient: The Consequences of Corporate Healthcare*. Munroe, ME: Common Courage Press, 2001.
18. Howe A. Written evidence from the Royal College of General Practitioners (CFI 30). House of Commons, 2011. https://publications.parliament.uk/pa/cm201011/cmselect/cmhealth/796/796vw31.htm (Accessed 4 March 2018).

19. NHS England. New models of care: Vanguards - developing a blueprint for the future of NHS and care services, 2016. https://www.england.nhs.uk/new-care-models/vanguards/care-models/community-sites/ (Accessed 4 March 2018).
20. NHS England. Five year forward view, 2014. https://www.england.nhs.uk/wp-content/uploads/2014/10/5yfv-web.pdf (Accessed 4 March 2018).
21. NHS England. Next steps on the five year forward view, 2017. https://www.england.nhs.uk/wp-content/uploads/2017/03/NEXT-STEPS-ON-THE-NHS-FIVE-YEAR-FORWARD-VIEW.pdf.
22. NHS England. Local partnerships to improve health and care. Sustainability and transformation partnerships (STPs) and integrated care systems (ICSs). NHS England, 2018. https://www.england.nhs.uk/system-change/ (Accessed 5 March 2018).
23. Charles A. Accountable care explained. Kings Fund, 2017. https://www.kingsfund.org.uk/publications/accountable-care-explained (Accessed 3 March 2018).
24. Salford Together. Sharing Medical and Care Records, 2016. http://www.salfordtogether.com/our_plans/sharing-medical-care-records/ (Accessed 4 March 2018).
25. Greater Manchester Academic Health Science Newtwork. Datawell Business Case. Delivering improved health and wellbeing by exchanging data, 2014. https://www.gmahsn.org/documents/23650/23814/GMAHSN+Datawell+Full+Business+Case.pdf/88087ced-20d0-409e-a37a-ddf-2739c4ca0 (Accessed 3 March 2018).
26. Connected Health Cities: University of Manchester, 2015. http://www.informatics.manchester.ac.uk/case-studies/connected-health-cities/ (Accessed 4 March 2018).

10.2 Achievements in East London

1. NHS Digital. Quality and outcomes framework. Quality and outcomes framework data 2016/17 results: 2017. http://qof.digital.nhs.uk/ (Accessed 3 April 2018).
2. Hull S, Chowdhury TA, Mathur R, Robson J. Improving outcomes for patients with type 2 diabetes using general practice networks: A quality improvement project in east London. *BMJ Qual Saf* 2014;23:171–176.
3. Robson J, Hull S, Mathur R, Boomla K. Improving cardiovascular disease using managed networks in general practice: An observational study in inner London. *Br J Gen Pract* 2014;64:e268–e274.
4. Robson J, Dostal I, Mathur R, Sohanpal R, Hull S, Antoniou S et al. Improving anticoagulation in atrial fibrillation: Observational study in three primary care trusts. *Br J Gen Pract* 2014;64:e275–e281.
5. Hull S, Mathur R, Lloyd-Owen S, Round T, Robson J. Improving outcomes for people with COPD by developing networks of general practices: Evaluation of a quality improvement project in East London. *NPJ Prim Care Respir Med* 2014;24:14082.

6. Cockman P, Dawson L, Mathur R, Hull S. Improving MMR vaccination rates: Herd immunity is a realistic goal. *BMJ* 2011;343:d5703.
7. Homer K, Robson J, Solaiman S, Davis A, Khan SZ, McCoy D et al. Reducing liver function tests for statin monitoring: An observational comparison of two clinical commissioning groups. *Br J Gen Pract* 2017;67:e194–e200.
8. Robson J, Smithers H, Chowdhury T, Bennett-Richards P, Keene D, Dostal I et al. Reduction in self-monitoring of blood glucose in type 2 diabetes: An observational controlled study in East London. *Br J Gen Pract* 2015;65:e256–e263.

10.3 Development in East London

1. Robson J. Statin guidance update: Clinical Effectiveness Group, 2015. https://www.qmul.ac.uk/blizard/media/blizard/documents/ceg-documents/Statin-Guidance-Update,-June-2015.pdf (Accessed 4 March 2018).
2. Clinical Effectiveness Group. CEG website. Queen Mary University of London: Centre for Primary Care and Public Health, 2018. https://www.qmul.ac.uk/blizard/ceg/resource-library/ (Accessed 4 March 2018).
3. Pawa J, Robson J, Hull S. Building managed primary care practice networks to deliver better clinical care: A qualitative semi-structured interview study. *Br J Gen Pract* 2017;67:e764–e774.
4. Michie S, van Stralen MM, West R. The behaviour change wheel: A new method for characterising and designing behaviour change interventions. *Implement Sci* 2011;6:42.
5. Dixon-Woods M, McNicol S, Martin G. Ten challenges in improving quality in healthcare: Lessons from the Health Foundation's programme evaluations and relevant literature. *BMJ Qual Saf* 2012;21:876–884.
6. Suter E, Oelke ND, Adair CE, Armitage GD. Ten key principles for successful health systems integration. *Healthc Q* 2009;13:16–23.
7. Bhatia RS, Levinson W, Shortt S, Pendrith C, Fric-Shamji E, Kallewaard M et al. Measuring the effect of Choosing Wisely: An integrated framework to assess campaign impact on low-value care. *BMJ Qual Saf* 2015;24:523–531.
8. Wallace E, Smith SM, Fahey T, Roland M. Reducing emergency admissions through community based interventions. *BMJ* 2016;352:h6817.
9. Zulman DM, Pal Chee C, Ezeji-Okoye SC, Shaw JG, Holmes TH, Kahn JS et al. Effect of an intensive outpatient program to augment primary care for high-need veterans affairs patients: A randomized clinical trial. *JAMA Intern Med* 2017;177:166–175.

10. McMurray JJ, Adamopoulos S, Anker SD, Auricchio A, Bohm M, Dickstein K et al. ESC Guidelines for the diagnosis and treatment of acute and chronic heart failure 2012: The Task Force for the Diagnosis and Treatment of Acute and Chronic Heart Failure 2012 of the European Society of Cardiology. Developed in collaboration with the Heart Failure Association (HFA) of the ESC. *Eur J Heart Fail* 2012;14:803–869.

11. Hotchkiss JW, Davies CA, Dundas R, Hawkins N, Jhund PS, Scholes S et al. Explaining trends in Scottish coronary heart disease mortality between 2000 and 2010 using IMPACTSEC model: Retrospective analysis using routine data. *BMJ* 2014;348:g1088.

12. Wachter RM. Making IT work: Harnessing the power of health information technology to improve care in England. Report of the National Advisory Group on Health Information Technology in England: National Advisory Group on Health Information Technology in England, 2016.

13. James BC, Savitz LA. How Intermountain trimmed health care costs through robust quality improvement efforts. *Health Aff (Millwood)* 2011;30:1185–1191.

14. Institute of Medicine (U.S.). Committee on Quality of Health Care in America. *Crossing the Quality Chasm: A New Health System for the 21st Century*. Washington, DC: National Academy Press, 2001.

15. Califf RM, Robb MA, Bindman AB, Briggs JP, Collins FS, Conway PH et al. Transforming evidence generation to support health and health care decisions. *N Engl J Med* 2016;375:2395–2400.

11

Core topics

The moral test of government is how that government treats those who are in the dawn of life, the children; those who are in the twilight of life, the elderly; and those who are in the shadows of life, the sick, the needy and the handicapped.

Hubert Humphrey
U.S. Senator

In the following sections, Professor Phil Wilson discusses the ways in which childhood predicts future physical and mental health and also the approaches that GPs can take to anticipate and avoid problems. Dr Anne Mullin follows by addressing the same issues from the perspective of a GP working in a very deprived area of Glasgow. Dr Andrea Williamson then addresses mental health issues in deprived areas and in particular the needs of people for whom mental distress is not a single problem requiring specialist treatment but part of a complex mix of physical, psychological and social issues. Dr Euan Paterson closes the section by considering end-of-life care.

11.1 THE DYNAMICS OF FAMILY LIFE

Although many health professions and services are concerned with children, general practice is unusual in its broad contact with families over long periods of time, as exemplified by the following anonymised vignette.

David is 14 months old. His 18-year-old mum, Sarah, has had anxiety problems since her older brother hanged himself four years ago. She started college but left when she fell pregnant shortly afterwards. Sarah does not get on well with her mother, whom she accuses of drinking and "always shouting" since her brother died. Her mum says she is "mental" and a "teenage brat". Sarah relies heavily on her own gran Margaret. Aged 50 she has moderately severe COPD (emphysema) and continues to smoke. Margaret has had several chest infections recently and is struggling to cope with Sarah's often strange behaviour and with a lively toddler for whom she is the main caregiver.

For David the next two years, as he learns to walk, talk and interact, will have a huge effect on the rest of his life. Early years interventions such as parenting classes may be important, but on their own will fail to change his life opportunities. He will need supportive neighbours, a good nursery and adequate family income, but also optimal COPD nurse reviews, responsive alcohol and mental health services, good communication with social work, persistent contraceptive advice and smoking cessation support, to name a few. At the hub of these lies the primary care team, offering unconditional care and the possibility of trusted relationships over the span of David's life.

Deep End Report 20 (1)

Parenting is a difficult job and even more challenging when parents have physical or mental health issues, their child has learning difficulties or refuses to attend school, the family has fled civil war in its native country or is overburdened with home-based or external stresses. Parents look to the state for support when times are difficult. That support may be from financial, educational, housing, employment or health services. Three centuries of sustained child welfare reform have underpinned this expectation, but there are worrying current trends.

Child poverty in the United Kingdom increased from 10% in 1979 to 30% in 1986. The children affected by this trend are now parents and have children of their own. Successive governments have tried to reduce the level of child poverty, with some progress during the period of Labour Government between 1997 and 2010. Since then, the figure has begun to increase and is forecast to reach 37% by 2022. In Scotland, there is no local authority with child poverty rates in single figures (2).

11.2 THE CHILD IN THE CONSULTING ROOM – WHAT DOES THE FUTURE HOLD?

PHIL WILSON

We regularly see adult patients with mental health problems, addictions or other health-harming behaviours, which seem to be rooted in an unhappy childhood. We sometimes ask ourselves whether things might have worked out better if we or others had been able to offer effective support at the first sign of things going wrong.

As GPs, we are used to integrating our knowledge of risk factors for morbidity and premature mortality and doing something about them. In recent years, GPs have focussed less on preventive child health and more on chronic disease management (1). As a consequence, we have tended to think less about the life-course perspective and more about the management of risk factors such as high blood pressure. But at a whole-population level, childhood risk factors are a far more potent source of premature mortality and morbidity than any physical examination finding.

11.2.1 Links between early adversity and adult health

Predisposing factors for poor mental and physical health later in life include:

- Genetic factors (e.g. vulnerability to ADHD or autism)
- Antenatal factors (e.g. maternal stress hormones, smoking and alcohol consumption)
- Factors located in the family/upbringing (e.g. postnatal depression, harsh or inconsistent parenting, parental discord)
- Factors located in the wider environment (e.g. relative poverty, neighbourhood problems)

These factors have been identified in many long-term studies (2) and interact in different ways. Some are additive, some multiplicative, while others may increase resilience to adversity, for example, there seem to be protective effects of high childhood verbal IQ and positive parent–infant interaction.

11.2.2 Genetic factors

Genetic factors have an impact on long-term physical and mental health, and sometimes we can take straightforward actions such as prescribing statins in familial hypercholesterolaemia. The impact of other inherited conditions is less simple, for example, ADHD which along with inattention and motor hyperactivity is associated with lack of impulse control, risk-taking behaviour, addictions and language disorders – all of which are associated with physical morbidity and/or premature mortality. We should pay attention to family histories of neurodevelopmental problems.

11.2.3 Antenatal factors

Teratogens such as valproate and alcohol can damage the growing fetus. It is less well known that high levels of maternal stress during pregnancy can have profound and permanent effects on the foetal brain through epigenetic influences. High levels of maternal circulating cortisol are amplified in the foetal circulation, causing methylation (and functional inactivation) of genes coding brain glucocorticoid receptors. The unborn child's hypothalamic-pituitary-adrenal axis is re-programmed, leading to altered stress responses (3).

As well as having direct adverse effects on foetal stress responses, maternal stress can disrupt the development of sensitivity to the unborn child. Antenatal depression is a stronger predictor of insensitive parenting (and, thus, childhood mental health problems) than postnatal depression (4).

11.2.4 Family factors

It is harder to provide a nurturing environment for a child when parents are stressed. Nevertheless, the relationship between parental mental state and parenting behaviours, particularly sensitivity to the child's needs, is not linear. All GPs have worked with profoundly depressed mothers who are excellent parents, and with perfectly mentally healthy parents who are insensitive to their infants' needs. Although parental emotional well-being is a major predictor of child development (5), parenting behaviours have a stronger influence (6,7).

In summary, there are strong but complex associations between parental mental health, parenting behaviours, children's brain development and, ultimately, adult health (8–11).

11.2.5 Environmental factors

Socio-demographic inequalities in early childhood mental health (12) are probably mediated by parental stress and other adverse childhood experiences such as abuse, neglect, family disruption, problem substance use, and so on. These inequalities are amplified in the first years of formal schooling (13), presumably because more privileged children are likely to thrive in the school environment whereas children without these advantages do not. Dealing with early childhood inequalities is an absolute prerequisite for reducing adult health inequalities. It is too late to leave it to adulthood (14).

11.2.6 How can we GPs identify childhood risk?

Although most brain development problems do not meet WHO criteria for screening programmes (there is little good research in this area), there are strong arguments for keeping a watchful eye on children's developmental vulnerability whenever the opportunity arises (15). Screening implies a single pass/fail test while surveillance implies a more continuous, nuanced approach designed to identify individuals at risk of a broad set of problems. The domains to which we should pay particular attention include:

- **Parental mental health:** Parents with mental health problems struggle to a greater or lesser extent to provide optimal care for their children. GPs should always ask how patients with psychiatric problems (including personality disorders) are getting on with their children and make their own observations whenever possible.
- **Parent–child interaction:** Positive parenting behaviours have an extremely strong protective effect against mental health problems in children (7), while negative parenting behaviours are likely to produce the opposite effect. We all have some degree of emotional reaction to positive or negative parent–child interactions in the consulting room but a more systematic approach to observation of the relationship can help, particularly when we need to communicate concerns to other professionals such as health visitors or social workers.

- **Child language**: Normal early language development requires adequate cognitive, sensory and motor functioning as well as sufficient opportunities to engage in verbal communication. There is some evidence for neurodevelopmental critical or sensitive periods in language acquisition. Normal language function is unlikely to be attained if there are physiological or social barriers to verbal communication in the early years. Impaired language acquisition is common and strongly associated with poor mental health in childhood and later life. Isolated language disorder is the exception rather than the rule.

  Delay in language acquisition is particularly strongly associated with ADHD, autism spectrum conditions, conduct disorder and severe attachment problems. Most children excluded from school and most young offenders have receptive language disorders and most of the psychiatric and behavioural problems that are co-morbid with language disorders are associated with a range of long-term pathologies. Demographic inequalities in language attainment are very obvious after age three years, and they closely mirror inequalities in health. Early language has been termed a "life chance indicator" and we should pay attention to it.

- **Child behaviour**: A child's behaviour in the consulting room can give important insights into what is going on in the child's relationships at home. A young child who is experiencing neglect may appear disengaged from social interaction or may seek attention in a strikingly disinhibited way. Indiscriminate friendliness and failure to seek proximity to a parent in a two- to three-year-old child can be an important sign of very dysfunctional attachment which bodes badly for the child's future. Similarly, very disruptive behaviour in the consulting room can indicate a range of problems which could be located in the child, the parents or the parent–child relationship. In the large 1958 UK birth cohort, children whose oppositional behaviour was rated in the upper quartile at age seven were twice as likely to have died by age 46 than those in the lower quartile (11).

11.2.7 What can we do when we find these risk factors?

As GPs, there is not a lot we can offer in terms of intensive therapeutic input when we suspect problems in child neurodevelopment, mental well-being or in the parent–child relationship, but we can do a lot in terms of early (opportunistic) identification and signposting towards useful services or onward referral (15) while maintaining a good ongoing therapeutic relationship with the family.

We are in an ideal position to challenge rigid institutional policies, when needed in the interests of the child, and to advocate for families when there are clear gaps in local service provision. This can be particularly powerful when we have longstanding knowledge of both the family and the locality. At the same time, we need to have good working relationships with those agencies that can offer support.

For GPs in the United Kingdom, maintaining a good working relationship with health visitors, ideally through regular face-to-face contact, is likely to be the most useful thing we can do for young children in our practice. Health visitors often have useful insights on the home environment and (particularly) mother–child relationships, while GPs often have complementary knowledge about the wider network of adults in the child's life and have the benefit of being able to observe parent–child relationships under the stressful circumstances surrounding illness.

11.3 LEVELLING UP IN DEEP END PRACTICES

ANNE MULLIN

The RCGP firmly believes that general practice occupies a central position in children and young people's health, particularly in the diagnosis and management of illness and the promotion of health and wellbeing. We are concerned that unless the profession acts now to protect this important and trusted role, it will become eroded and lead to serious fragmentation of care for this vulnerable group of patients. (1)

11.3.1 More than skin deep

According to the RCGP Child Health Strategy, GPs should be involved in all aspects of maintaining child health and well-being. This will not surprise GPs who understand their role as family doctors, treat members of the same family and can witness the distress that is described in the vignette above (Section 11.1). 'David', 'Sarah' and 'Margaret' will all consult with their GP over their lifetimes and it is the GP who is often the constant professional in their lives. 'David' will eventually no longer require health visitor input as he enters school, 'Sarah's' anxiety will probably not require long-term support from mental health services and 'Margaret' will be discharged by the respiratory clinic, but all will meet the criteria for unconditional continuity of care that is provided by their GP.

The GP as a 'trusted ally' (2) has an important advocacy role for vulnerable families in encouraging them to engage with supportive services. A non-judgemental approach by an experienced GP who has cumulative knowledge of family function can make a positive difference to family outcomes particularly in situations where child safeguarding concerns do not meet the thresholds of statutory intervention.

Deep End GPs, in particular, 'are well placed to understand the specific challenges that result in the vulnerable family and the vulnerable child and have an important role to play in contributing to the mitigation and reduction of inequities in health' (3). It is puzzling, therefore, that the role of the generalist in addressing the complexity of family health and well-being is not always clearly written into policies for child health.

For example, Scotland's national child safeguarding policy GIRFEC (Getting It Right For Every Child) does not specify the role of the GP (4), with the result that other agencies may not recognise the role of GPs when the policy is put into effect. General practice is then written out of the narrative of child health and well-being, with a consequent diminution of preventative child health care (5).

GPs have an intuitive grasp of identifying children 'in need' during clinical contacts with vulnerable families (6). Parental mental health problems and addictions, for example, allow GPs to identify such a child during the 'indirect consultation'. The vignette at the start of this Section provides a snapshot of such a family that is struggling with the effects of household dysfunction and adverse childhood experiences (ACEs).

GPs are pragmatic problem solvers and well-placed to instigate and coordinate practical measures to help de-stress families and foster their resilience. The vignette is not written from a distance but from the proximity of a holistic practitioner with in-depth, experiential knowledge of his patients and using this knowledge, not to police or judge but to support and ameliorate suffering in a family that has multiple unmet needs. This is the essence of working in general practice with vulnerable children and families (7).

11.3.2 It's taking quite a long time – Why are poor children still with us?

In a country where the income and wealth gaps have become greater than at any point in living memory, and which are greater than in almost all other similar wealthy countries, you should expect very high and rising levels of crime, social disorder, dysfunction, rising polarisation, fear and anxiety.

Danny Dorling (8)

Poverty and its effects on child health are persistent, historic and dependent on the political ideologies and state responses that alleviate or exacerbate the extent and depth of poverty. The many services including general practice that provide support to vulnerable families and children should consider the effects of poverty when exploring family dysfunction and child maltreatment (9).

It is striking that doctors working in the NHS today are voicing similar concerns about the lasting effects of child poverty as those made by doctors in earlier times.

'Doctors explained that they have seen a combination of increasing poverty and housing problems, and cuts to other services which have left families with less support, such as parenting guidance, children's centres, speech and language and other therapies, youth provision, opportunities for exercise and stress relief, and services for disabled children.

Equal access to health services is an important leveller. Better-off families may be able to access these services privately or drive to reach them, but low-income families may simply be left behind' (10).

The burden of inequality rests mostly on the shoulders of young people who bear the brunt of toxic policies that marginalise them and 'pathologise poverty'. Current UK welfare policies are reversing decades of progressive child welfare reforms that have always been highly contingent on local and national conditions (11).

Far from being peripheral to this debate, the medical profession is inextricably linked to the politics of child welfare and child poverty (12).

GPs are not short of reference material in all matters of child health and well-being. Some answers will reside in the churn of documents that are updated or renewed on an annual basis but despite an expansive evidence base on the effects of child poverty on child health and well-being, the GP contribution to the issue has been variable and inconsistent.

Which lens gives the clearest vision of the GP role in preventing the adverse effects of toxic stress in childhood? The profession as a whole seems to have a blind spot. Working in a Deep End practice can foster empathy with the plight of impoverished patients but GPs could do much more, especially by adding their 'powerful voices' to political concerns (13).

11.3.3 Seeing 'stuff' through an ACE's lens

I've only seen the term 'ACE' relatively recently (mainly, in fact, through stuff you've sent out to us over past couple of years re children/poverty etc). The stuff though not very surprising seems so relevant to work with Deep End populations

Personal email from Deep End GP

Certain periods of time mark a progression in society's approach to child welfare issues. Scotland is developing its own response to the challenges of health inequalities by prioritising the negative health effects of child poverty and adverse childhood events (ACEs) (14). Both are high on the policy agenda and recognised as problems for society to address.

The ACE lens provides an alternative way of understanding adversity in childhood and family dysfunction, which have previously tended to feature mainly within accounts of child maltreatment (15) and which have, therefore, been under-reported.

ACEs are common factors that have an impact on parenting, increasing family dysfunction and stress. From a landmark retrospective epidemiological study in the United States, 10 distressing experiences within the family setting were identified (16).

- Domestic violence
- Emotional neglect
- Physical abuse
- Sexual abuse
- Parental separation
- Alcohol misuse
- Drug misuse
- Mental illness
- Suicide
- Imprisonment of a member of the household

The study showed clear cumulative correlations with negative adult physical and mental health outcomes across the lifespan. The findings have been confirmed in UK populations (17).

GPs now have reference points with which to understand the antecedents that predict poor adult health and well-being and which make sense in everyday family GP contacts. With this information, general practice can progress beyond its marginal involvement in policies addressing the key social issues that influence risky health behaviours, multimorbidity, end of healthy life expectancy and early mortality.

It is tempting to foresee that an ACE-informed workforce may solve the perennial problem of identifying the unmet need in vulnerable families but there are important caveats, as the ten conventional ACEs may not be sufficient to encapsulate all significant adversity. There is significant overlap between the effects of current ACEs and poverty (which is not included in the ACEs list) on internal family stresses (18).

Higher family income is not always a protective factor (19). Any suggestion that widespread screening for ACEs can substitute for watchful waiting and pragmatic intervention should be considered with caution. GPs will have difficulty in formalising ACEs prevention during a busy working day when there may be many reasons for reluctance to ask a patient about childhood experiences, including professional inexperience, personal beliefs, relevance to clinical presentations and impact on health matters (20).

Child neglect and abuse are uncomfortable terms for many practitioners, and thresholds for child protection procedures are not the metric that will determine the scale of unmet need in vulnerable children. ACEs offer an alternative and expansive language that is more suited to holistic family medicine and not the formality of restrictive child protection measures. An ACEs-informed narrative that is developed through routine inquiry (21) can support a more humanitarian and nurturing approach to the complex stresses and interactions that define family life.

11.3.4 Small Lives, Small Data – Govan SHIP

General practice is perceived as being 'not child-friendly' (22). A supportive working environment for GPs should be a priority to overcome professional apathy or negative attitudes about working with vulnerable families but will not happen spontaneously. This work requires governmental aspirational policies and committed professionals in primary care with an adequate resource to undertake what is often time-consuming work to foster resilience in families. However, there is an economic benefit to society in the cost savings associated with primary prevention (23). If it remains under-resourced and fragmented, general practice will be left with the dilemma of finding time to work with families who have multiple vulnerability factors and present during a busy working day seeking help and support. With its intrinsic contact, continuity and coverage, general practice is the natural hub for local health systems and working alongside partner agencies can build community resilience (24) and maximise strengths and minimise weaknesses in complex family lives (25).

The Govan Social Healthcare Integrated Project (SHIP) shows the potential of such a service where GPs are given protected time to directly engage with vulnerable children and families and plan comprehensive support plans during a monthly multidisciplinary team (MDT) meeting (Section 7.1). The MDT may result in referral to the health visitor, engaging with educational support or child mental health services or providing additional parental supports. It may require one or all of these approaches as each individual situation demands a unique response (26). At the core of this work is a child-focused general practice that is integrated with partner agencies and working beyond a 'mandate' of child protection (27). It does not require the evangelisation or commodification of ACEs but a holistic and pragmatic general practice approach that has always, it seems, understood supportive working with the vulnerable family when left to practise the art and science of the day job.

11.4 MENTAL HEALTH

ANDREA WILLIAMSON

Deep End GPs work with communities in Scotland with high and often extreme socioeconomic deprivation (1). The following text is drawn from Deep End Reports 22 and 26 on mental health in deprived areas and calls for a more patient-centred approach and better integration of services.

11.4.1 Context

Communities experiencing high socioeconomic deprivation have to cope with disproportionately negative social determinants of health and resultant mental health difficulties despite resilience factors being present (2,3).

Measurable mental ill health is twice as prevalent in socioeconomically deprived areas as in affluent areas (4). It is the most common comorbidity in deprived communities. The prevalence of mental ill health increases in direct proportion to the number of other problems a person has (5).

Such patients need integrated care, not the separation of the mental health component by stand-alone services.

The patients with the lowest enablement scores after seeing their GP are those with mental health problems in socioeconomically deprived areas (6–8) – a symptom of how general practice is struggling to work effectively in this context. The high prevalence of long-term antidepressant prescribing is another indicator of how general practice struggles to respond and cope (9) in the context of constrained resources (10).

11.4.2 Concepts

Psychological distress is a more effective basis for the framing of patient care needs than diagnostic categories – which, from a general practice perspective, tend to screen people out rather than include people in. This is especially true of crisis, out of hours and community mental health services, which are experienced by many patients and perceived by GPs as trying to find ways not to provide support.

"Psychological distress" takes account of patients' experience. People experience symptoms rather than a diagnostic label.

Greater recognition should be given to the effect that complex trauma and adverse childhood experiences (Section 11.3) have on mental ill health across the whole Scottish population (11,12) but especially in communities with higher levels of adversity.

This should be recognised and responded to by:

- A continued focus on prevention in the early years and with families.
- By embedding trauma-informed practice (13) and mentalising skills (14) in all mental health services – rather than in pockets of good practice.
- Problem substance use (including alcohol) should be reframed as "escape coping" (using substances to block memories, emotions or manage symptoms) rather than a problem separate from patients who experience mental health difficulties.
- Service design and evaluation should be culturally sensitive (15) especially for people with low engagement patterns with care, including specific consideration for people who are marginalised such as being homeless or a recent migrant (Chapter 12).
- There should be a focus on better understanding of resilience and vulnerability, in the short and longer terms, over a person's life course. This is in order to target episodic versus ongoing support needs so that patients experience continuity of care from the professionals around them.

11.4.3 Service structure

Solutions need to pay attention to the current large gaps experienced by patients and primary care professionals seeking to support patients with substance-use problems and mental health symptoms. Both systems provide good quality care – but in silos – and this leads to patients with complex needs falling between the cracks and often experiencing very poor outcomes (16).

Recognition is needed that mental health functioning has an impact on patient's ability to engage with all health care including physical health concerns. Multimorbidity is the norm for most patients with mental health difficulties. The health service should be structured around patients' needs rather than the need of the health service to work in professional and disciplinary silos.

A reframing of services around the complexity of needs (including physical needs) would be an effective way of re-organising mental health services away from diagnostic categories (for example, work on supporting patients who experience severe and multiple disadvantages) (17).

A key way to support this would be to co-locate mental health services within general practice clusters and provide attached mental health workers to work flexibly within practices. This works better not only for patients but also for professionals – better relationships, communication, continuity, and better use of community resources (18).

Shared records between mental health services, general practice and social work should support this development.

11.4.4 Attached complex needs mental health workers

Attached complex needs MH workers should engage and collaborate with community and specialist mental health services in adult and children's services to improve communication and joint working – this is a specific request for an attached MH worker, not necessarily a community psychiatric nurse (CPN) (19). The MH worker would attend primary care/GP MDT meetings to discuss caseloads and patients' unmet needs with the extended primary care team, matching mental health care at the right level based on their needs. This may involve statutory mental health services or third-sector agencies (20).

11.4.5 Patient and community focus

Without detracting from the important contribution that mental health professionals make towards the support of patients experiencing mental distress, the role that other public sector organisations and community-based organisations have in supporting patients when in crisis, recovering or thriving should be recognised and supported.

We would like to see shared learning opportunities across mental health services, general practice and third-sector-based organisations to promote shared decision making and inter-professional collaboration (21). This would enhance everyone's professional practice (22).

A useful way to broker more effective community involvement would be the rolling out of the link worker model (23,24) to include mental health services within primary care clusters.

The NHS Health Scotland evaluation of the Link Worker programme showed that patients engaging with link workers had better outcomes with respect to ill health, anxiety, depression, isolation, smoking and employment (25,26). Although the programme had no defined entry criteria and the evaluation was not a randomised controlled trial, the results suggest that there are levels of poor mental health in the community, which may not meet thresholds for referral or evidence-based treatment but which can be improved by a prompt, unconditional approach to patients' problems in a familiar setting with a professional person they know and trust.

Mental health services would then be better placed to support patients across the full spectrum of mental health needs in conjunction with access to public sector and voluntary sector support for other needs such as housing and benefits.*

* See also Section 9.4 on Community Practice linking community services for physical and mental health in Pittsburgh, Pennsylvania.

11.5 END-OF-LIFE CARE

EUAN PATERSON

To be with people at the edge of the human predicament, to understand them when they were there and, to some extent, to let them understand me being with them at that point.

Kieran Sweeney (1)

There could be no better introduction to this section on palliative and end-of-life care than Professor Kieran Sweeney's description of his role as the doctor. The palliative care that a GP provides is simply good care for people who are dying, and thus the aspects of the GP's role outlined in this section are applicable in all situations that the GP encounters. However, the enormity of death and the surrounding emotional issues mean that care at this stage of the patient's life is sometimes the most important care that a GP can provide.

Providing compassionate palliative care, based on an empathetic recognition of the patient's situation and coupled with a desire to relieve their suffering, has not only obvious significant benefits for the patient and their loved ones but also provides GPs with some of the most powerful professional satisfaction that they will encounter.

Caring for the dying patient and those close to them presents the GP with the opportunity to demonstrate the synthesis of the treating and healing roles of their profession by providing care that is both transactional and relational.

The elements of good transactional care are perhaps easier to define. This is the domain of technical competence where the science of medicine is found. The knowledge and skills derived from at least nine years of undergraduate and post-graduate training, coupled with the experience of the complexity of GP practice, make the GP the most competent diagnostician in the primary care team.

In this context diagnosis encompasses not only major conditions such as heart failure or cancer but also the myriad of smaller but critical diagnoses, each an arrival at some point of relative clarity – the cause of a symptom, the level of support required, how much of the dying person's resilience is left – an almost endless list of vital decision points. In addition, it will usually be the GP who makes the critical diagnosis of 'dying' – the hard to define point where the aim of care must start to include a good and dignified death along with disease amelioration, improvement and survival.

In every encounter, countless such diagnoses are reached. And for each of these, some form of treatment plan has to be considered. Issues include where it is safe for the patient to be, should admission be offered, what medications might help, what additional support is offered and, of course, when review of each and every one of these should occur.

Closely linked to the above, and again due to training and clinical experience, the GP is likely to be seen as the senior clinical decision maker within the primary care team. This role takes the GP into some very deep and complex issues. Though it is essential to involve patients in any decision that concerns their well-being, initial decisions around what to offer people will frequently be taken by the GP. The most obvious example of this are decisions relating to cardiopulmonary resuscitation (CPR). In most palliative care situations, the GP will decide clinically whether their patient should or should not be offered CPR. This decision must then be presented to and discussed with the patient. This is not just the case for CPR decisions. In many situations, it is incumbent on the GPs to decide what they believe offers the best outcome for the patient and then discuss the pros and cons of this potential course of action with the individual before arriving at the course of action that the patient feels is most suitable.

The GP also has a key role in endorsing or ratifying the decisions of others. Most importantly these will be decisions arrived at by the patient. A dying patient who states that they do not wish CPR would have this decision endorsed and documented by their GP. The GP will also ratify, and thus take responsibility for, decisions made by other team members, for example, acting on the suggestion of the District Nurse to prescribe Just in Case anticipatory medication, laxatives or skin care preparations.

In palliative care, and indeed in all aspects of care, the GP is in the unique position of having a significant pre-morbid awareness of their patient. This ability to hold a biography of the patient is born out of the narrative supplied by serial encounters, often over many years. This is vitally important to the treatment aspects of the GP role outlined above enabling the GP to deal with the utterly undifferentiated presentation and to seek out, with the patient, what matters in a vast bio-psycho-social-spiritual arena. These are consultations where context, past behaviours and deep mutual awareness all have their place alongside the explicit presentation.

It is this long-term relationship, where the GP is aware of what is important to the patient not only physically but in a social and spiritual context, that underpins the GP's significant healing roles in palliative care. These are part of the 'essence' of general practice and as such should be part of all good care but perhaps nowhere more important than in palliative and end-of-life care when the patient's death is looming.

Explanation is a key role of the GP in palliative care. It is important that the GP makes clear to the patient what is causing their symptoms, what can be offered and what outcomes are likely, which in this context includes the inevitability of death. The bad news is always bad news but if it is delivered compassionately within a relationship where both parties understand and trust each other it will be less burdensome for the patient. In addition, explanation can help to normalise some of what the person is experiencing. An example is acute grief – the person will expect to feel unhappy, sad, anxious, perhaps angry but explaining and normalising the unexpected physicality of grief will go a long way to ease suffering.

As potentially the patient's most trusted health care professional the GP is ideally placed to both affirm and validate the patient's views and beliefs. An increasingly topical example might be the patient who asks about a 'flight to Switzerland'. Acknowledging that the patient has simply had enough and validating the reasoning that has taken them to that point – even if one disagrees – will allow further dialogue and may well diminish any risk. A statement such as 'I can see how you might feel like that' could be the very support the patient requires to ease their burden – the parallel of asking the depressed patient about self-harm diminishing the likelihood of suicide.

The combination of explaining, normalising, validating and affirming helps the patient make sense of things, affording the opportunity of deeper understanding. This is perhaps best described by Peter Toon (2):

> The consultation is the patient's forum for coming to understand her illness; not merely a rational understanding, but an understanding that involves the emotions and which contributes to the growth of the individual.

The 'simple' support offered by the GP can be invaluable. For the GP to highlight the immense strength and courage that the patient has shown to come through their travail – the worry around diagnosis, the misery of treatment, their almost inevitable decline, the fear for those they will leave behind – is extremely therapeutic and, by extension, empowering.

Finally, one of the GP's most important functions is as a witness to the patient's suffering. This role is perhaps at its most powerful in palliative and end-of-life care. When modern medicine, despite its vast technical advances, has been unable to prevent disease progression or provide cure, there is an implicit admission from the GP of medicine's, and, by extension, their own technical shortcomings. The willingness of the GP, despite their 'fallibility', to simply be with their patient in their time of need is one of the GP's most compassionate acts.

In 'A Fortunate Man', arguably the best account of general practice, John Berger encapsulates the profound human need for relational care (3).

> He (Sassall) is acknowledged as a good doctor because he meets the deep but unformulated expectation of the sick for a sense of fraternity.

It is difficult to see where this sense of fraternity, the essence of general practice, could be of more value than when caring for the dying.

REFERENCES

11.1 The dynamics of family life

1. General Practitioners at the Deep End. Deep End Report 20: What can NHS Scotland do to prevent and reduce health inequalities? Proposals from General Practitioners at the Deep End. April 2013 www.gla.ac.uk/deepend.
2. End Child Poverty 2018. www.endchildpoverty.org.uk/poverty-in-your-area-2018.

11.2 The child in the consulting room – What does the future hold?

1. Wood R, Wilson P. General practitioner provision of preventive child health care: Analysis of routine consultation data. *BMC Family Practice* 2012;13:73.
2. Thompson L, Kemp J, Wilson P, Pritchett R, Minnis H, Toms-Whittle L, Puckering C, Law J, Gillberg C. What have birth cohort studies asked about genetic, pre- and peri-natal exposures and child and adolescent onset mental health outcomes? A systematic review. *European Child & Adolescent Psychiatry* 2010;19:1–15.
3. Hunter AL, Minnis H, Wilson P. Altered stress responses in children exposed to early adversity: A systematic review of salivary cortisol studies. *Stress* 2011;14(6):14–26. doi:10.3109/10253890.2011.577848.
4. Pearson RM, Melotti R, Heron J, Joinson C, Stein A, Ramchandani PG, Evans J. Disruption to the development of maternal responsiveness? The impact of prenatal depression on mother-infant interactions. *Infant Behavior and Development* 2012;35(4):613–626.
5. Tough SC, Siever JE, Leew S, Johnston DW, Benzies K, Clark D. Maternal mental health predicts risk of developmental problems at 3 years of age: Follow up of a community based trial. *BMC Pregnancy Childbirth* 2008;8(16):1–11.
6. Murray L, Hipwell A, Hooper R, Stein A, Cooper P. The cognitive development of 5-year-old children of postnatally depressed mothers. *Journal of Child Psychology & Psychiatry & Allied Disciplines* 1996;37(8):927–935.
7. Puckering C, Allely C, Doolin O, Purves D, McConnachie A, Johnson P, Marwick H et al. Association between parent-infant interactions in infancy and disruptive behaviour disorders at age seven: A nested, case-control ALSPAC study. *BMC Pediatrics* 2014;14(1):223. doi:10.1186/1471-2431-14-223.
8. Wilson P, Bradshaw P, Tipping S, Henderson M, Der G, Minnis H. What predicts persistent early conduct problems? Evidence from the growing up in Scotland cohort. *Journal of Epidemiology and Community Health* 2013;67(1):76–80.
9. Scott S, Lewsey J, Thompson L, Wilson P. Early parental physical punishment and emotional and behavioural outcomes in preschool children. *Child: Care, Health and Development* 2014;40(3):337–345.
10. Jokela M, Batty GD, Deary IJ, Gale CR, Kivimäki M. Low childhood IQ and early adult mortality: The role of explanatory factors in the 1958 British Birth Cohort. *Pediatrics* 2009;124(3):e380–e388.
11. Jokela M, Ferrie J, Kivimäki M. Childhood problem behaviors and death by midlife: The British national child development study. *Journal of the American Academy of Child & Adolescent Psychiatry* 2009;48(1):19–24.
12. Barry SJE, Marryat L, Thompson L, Ellaway A, White J, McClung M, Wilson P. Mapping area variability in social and behavioural difficulties among Glasgow pre-schoolers: Linkage of a survey of pre-school staff with routine monitoring data. *Child: Care, Health and Development* 2015;41(6):853–864.

13. Marryat L, Thompson L, Minnis H, Wilson P. Primary schools and the amplification of social differences in child mental health: A population-based cohort study. *Journal of Epidemiology and Community Health* 2018;72(1):27–33.doi:10.1136/jech-2017-208995.
14. Marmot M, Allen J, Goldblatt P, Boyce T, McNeish D, Grady M, Geddes I. *Fair Society, Healthy Lives: The Marmot Review.* London, UK: Department of Health, 2010.
15. Wilson P, Wood R, Lykke K, Hauskov Graungaard A, Ertmann RK, Andersen MK, Haavet OR et al. International variation in programmes for assessment of children's neurodevelopment in the community: Understanding disparate approaches to evaluation of motor, social, emotional, behavioural and cognitive function. *Scandinavian Journal of Public Health* 2018; 1403494818772211. doi:10.1177/1403494818772211.

11.3 Levelling up in Deep End practices

1. RCGP. RCGP Child Health Strategy 2010-2015. Internet. 1-1-2010. 3-1-0018.
2. Woodman J, Rafi I, de, LS. Child maltreatment: Time to rethink the role of general practice. *British Journal of General Practice* 2014;64(626):444–445.
3. GPs at the Deep End. Deep End Report 23. The contribution of general practice to improving the health of vulnerable children and families. June 2014. www.gla.ac.uk/deepend.
4. Coles E, Cheyne H, Rankin J, Daniel B. Getting it right for every child: A national policy framework to promote children's well-being in Scotland, United Kingdom. *The Milbank Quarterly* 2016;94(2):334–365.
5. Wood R, Wilson P. General practitioner provision of preventive child health care: Analysis of routine consultation data. *BMC Family Practice* 2012;13:73.
6. Lykke K, Christensen P, Reventlow S. The consultation as an interpretive dialogue about the child's health needs. *Family Practice* 2011;28(4):430–436. doi.org/10.1093/fampra/cmq111.
7. Gillies JC, Mercer SW, Lyon A, Scott M, Watt GCM. Distilling the essence of general practice: A learning journey in progress. *British Journal of General Practice* 2009;59(562):e167–e176.
8. Dorling D. The case for austerity among the rich. IPPR Discussion Paper on promoting growth and shared prosperity in the UK. Google. 1-1-2012. London, UK: Institute for Public Policy Research, 2018.
9. Featherstone B, Morris K, Daniel B, Bywaters P, Brady G, Bunting L, Mason W, Mirza N. Poverty, inequality, child abuse and neglect: Changing the conversation across the UK in child protection? *Children and Youth Services Review* 2017. Available from: http://www.sciencedirect.com/science/article/pii/S0190740917304425.

10. RCPCH. Poverty and children's health: Views from the frontline. RCPCH, 1 May 2015.
11. Blackman S. Rodgers R. *Youth Marginality In Britain: Contemporary Studies of Austerity.* Bristol, UK: Policy Press.
12. Watt G. On behalf of the Deep End Steering Group. Working with vulnerable families in deprived areas. *British Journal of General Practice* 2011;61(585):298.
13. Babbel B, Mackenzie M, Hastings A, Watt G. How do general practitioners understand health inequalities and do their professional roles offer scope for mitigation? Constructions derived from the Deep End of primary care. *Critical Public Health* 2017; 1–13.doi:10.1080/09581596.2017.1418499.
14. Scottish Public Health Network (ScotPHN). 'Polishing the Diamonds' Addressing Adverse Childhood Experiences in Scotland. Internet, 2016.
15. Reichman NE, Corman H, Noonan K, Jimenez ME. Infant health and future childhood adversity. *Maternal and Child Health Journal* 2018;22(3):318–326. doi:10.1007/s10995-017-24118-5.
16. Felitti VJ, Anda RF, Nordenberg D, Williamson DF, Spitz AM, Edwards V, Koss MP, Marks JS. Relationship of childhood abuse and household dysfunction to many of the leading causes of death in adults. The Adverse Childhood Experiences (ACE) Study. *American Journal of Preventive Medicine* 1998;14(4):245–258. doi:10.1016/S0749-3797(98)00017-8.
17. Hughes K, Bellis MA, Hardcastle KA, Sethi D, Butchart A, Mikton C, Jones L, Dunne MP. The effect of multiple adverse childhood experiences on health: A systematic review and meta-analysis. *Lancet Public Health* 2017;2(8):e356–e366. doi:10.1016/S2468-2667(17)30118-4.
18. Lanier P, Maguire-Jack K, Lombardi B, Frey J, Rose RA. Adverse childhood experiences and child health outcomes: Comparing cumulative risk and latent class approaches. *Maternal and Child Health Journal* 2018;22(3):288–297. doi:10.1007/s10995-017-2365-1.
19. Halfon N, Larson K, Son J, Lu M, Bethell C. Income inequality and the differential effect of adverse childhood experiences in US children. *Academic Pediatrics* 2017;17(7S):S70–S78. doi:10.1016/j.acap.2016.11.007.
20. Kerker BD, Storfer-Isser A, Szilagyi M, Stein RE, Garner AS, O'Connor KG, Hoagwood KE, Horwitz SM. Do pediatricians ask about adverse childhood experiences in pediatric primary care? *Academic Pediatrics* 2016;16(2):154–160. doi:10.1016/j.acap.2015.08.002.
21. NHS Health Scotland. Ace Routine Enquiry. 2017 Presentations. Available from http://www.healthscotland.scot/publications/aces-routine-enquiry-presentations.
22. Lang D. Letter-Response to 'How to protect general practice from child protection'. *British Journal of General Practice* 2011;61(586):326.
23. Steverman SM, Shern DL. Financing mechanisms for reducing adversity and enhancing resilience through implementation of primary prevention. *Academic Pediatrics* 2017;17(7S):S144–S149. doi:10.1016/j.acap.2017.04.003.

24. Ellis WR, Dietz WH. A new framework for addressing adverse child-hood and community experiences: The building community resilience model. *Academic Pediatrics* 2017;17(7S):S86–S93. doi:10.1016/j.acap.2016.12.011.

25. Ungar M. The differential impact of social services on young people's resilience. *Child Abuse & Neglect* 2018;78:4–12. doi:10.1016/j.chiabu.2017.09.024.

26. GPs at the Deep End. Deep End REPORT 29. GP use of additional time as part of the SHIP Project. www.gla.ac.uk/deepend, 2016.

27. Alberth L, Bühler-Niederberger D. Invisible children? Professional bricolage in child protection. *Children and Youth Services Review* 2015;57:149–158.

11.4 Mental health

1. Watt G. The Inverse Care Law today. *Lancet* 2002;360:252–254. doi:10.1016/S0140-6736(02)09466-7.

2. Dowrick C, Bower P, Chew-Graham C, Lovell K, Edwards S, Lamb J, Bristow K et al. Evaluating a complex model designed to increase access to high quality primary mental health care for under-served groups: A multi-method study. *BMC Health Services Research* 2016;16:58. doi:10.1186/s12913-016-1298-5.

3. Lamb J, Bower P, Rogers A, Dowrick C, Gask L. Access to mental health in primary care: A qualitative meta-synthesis of evidence from the experience of people from 'hard to reach' groups. *Health (London)* 2012;16(1):76–104.

4. Barnett K, Mercer SW, Norbury M, Watt G, Wyke S, Guthrie B. Epidemiology of multimorbidity and implications for health care, research, and medical education: A cross-sectional study. *Lancet* 2012; 380(9836):37–43. doi:10.1016/S0140-6736(12)60240-2.

5. Mclean G, Gunn J, Guthrie B, Watt GCM, Blane DN, Mercer SW. The influence of socioeconomic deprivation on multimorbidity at different ages. *British Journal of General Practice* 2014;64(624):e440–e447.

6. Mercer SW, Watt GCM. The Inverse Care Law: Clinical primary care encounters in deprived and affluent areas of Scotland. *Annals of Family Medicine* 2007;5:503–510. doi:10.1136/bmj.e4152.

7. Bhautesh J, Bikker AP, Higgins M, Fitzpatrick B, Little P, Watt GCM, Mercer SW. Patient centredness and the outcome of primary care consultations with patients with depression in areas of high and low socioeconomic deprivation. *British Journal of General Practice* 2012;62:e576–e581.

8. Mercer S, Higgins M, Bikker A, Fitzpatrick B, McConnachie A, Lloyd S, Little P, Watt GCM. General practitioner's empathy and health outcomes: A prospective observational study of consultations in areas of high and low deprivation. *Annals of Family Medicine* 2016;14:117–124. doi: 10.1370/afm.1910.

9. Tomlinson J, Mackay D, Watt G, Whyte B, Hanlon P, Tannahill C. The shape of primary care in NHS greater Glasgow and Clyde. *Glasgow Centre for Population Health* 2008. www.gcph.co.uk/component/option, com_docman/task, cat_view/gid,67/Itemid,71/.

10. McLean G, Guthrie B, Mercer SW, Watt GCM. General practice funding underpins the persistence of the Inverse Care Law: Cross-sectional study in Scotland. *British Journal of General Practice* 2015;v65(641):e799–805.

11. Shonkoff JP, Garner AS, The lifelong effects of early childhood adversity and toxic stress. *Pediatrics* 2014;36(2):102–108. doi:10.1542/peds.2011-2663.

12. Bellis M. Lowey H, Leckenby N, Hughes K, Harrison D. Adverse childhood experiences: Retrospective study to determine their impact on adult health behaviours and health outcomes in a UK population. *Journal of Public Health* 2014:36:81–91. doi:10.1093?pubmed/fdt038.

13. BC Provincial Mental Health and Substance Use Planning Council. Trauma informed practice guide. British Columbia, Canada, 2013. Available from http://bccewh.bc.ca/publications-resources/documents/TIP-Guide-May2013.pdf.

14. Homelessness and Personality Disorder Team, Case Study, Glasgow. Available from http://blogs.iriss.org.uk/homelessness/personality-disorder/.

15. Lovell K, Lamb J, Gask L, Bower P, Waheed W, Chew-Graham C, Lamb J et al. Development and evaluation of culturally sensitive psychosocial interventions for under-served people in primary care. *BMC Psychiatry* 2014;14:217.

16. Mental Health in Scotland- closing the gaps making a difference. 2007. Available from http://www.gov.scot/Resource/Doc/206410/0054849.pdf.

17. Lankelly Chase. Severe and Multiple Disadvantage Theory of Change. Available from http://lankellychase.org.uk/multiple- disadvantage/.

18. Railton S, Mowat H, and Bain J. Optimizing the care of patients with depression in primary care: The views of general practitioners. *Health & Social Care in the Community* 2000;8(2):119–128.

19. Simmons MB, Hetrick SE, Jorm AF. Making decisions about treatment for young people diagnosed with depressive disorders: A qualitative study of clinicians' experiences. *BMC Psychiatry* 2013;13:335.

20. Agius M, Murphy CL, Zaman R. Does shared care help in the treatment of depression? *Psychiatria Danubina* 2010;22 Suppl 1:S18–S22.

21. Chong WW, Aslani P, Chen TF. Shared decision-making and interprofessional collaboration in mental healthcare: A qualitative study exploring perceptions of barriers and facilitators. *Journal of Interprofessional Care* 2013;27(5):373–379.

22. Coupe N, Anderson E, Gask L, Sykes P, Richards DA, Chew-Graham C. Facilitating professional liaison in collaborative care for depression in UK primary care; a qualitative study utilising normalisation process theory. *BMC Family Practice* 2014;15:78. doi:10.1186/1471-2296-15-78.

23. Mossabir R, Morris R, Kennedy A, Blickem C, Rogers A. A scoping review to understand the effectiveness of linking schemes from healthcare providers to community resources to improve the health and well-being of people with long-term conditions. *Health & Social Care in the Community* 2015;23:467–484. doi:10.1111/hsc.12176.
24. National Links Worker Programme Records of Learning. Available from http://www.alliance-scotland.org.uk/resources/library/grid/1/type/all/topic/13/tag/all/condition/all/page/.
25. Mercer SW, Fitzpatrick B, Grant L, Rui Chng N, O'Donnell CA, Mackenzie M, McConnachie A, Bakhshi A, Wyke S. The Glasgow 'Deep End' Links Worker Study: Protocol of a quasi-experimental evaluation of a social prescribing complex intervention for patients with multiple complex needs in areas of high socioeconomic deprivation. *Journal of Comorbidity* 2017;7:1–10.
26. NHS Health Scotland. Evaluation of the Glasgow "Deep End" Links Worker Programme. NHS Health Scotland, 2017 http://www.healthscotland.scot/publications/evaluation-of-the-linksworker-programme-in-deep-end-general-practices-in-glasgow.

11.5 End-of-life care

1. Sweeney K. Interview. Available from https://www.youtube.com/watch?v=3TignNvHNx4
2. Toon P. What is good general practice? Occasional Paper 65. Exeter: RCGP, 1994.
3. Berger J, Mohr J. *A Fortunate Man – The Story of a Country Doctor.* London, UK: Allen Lane, Penguin Press 1967.

12

Learning from medicine at the margins

Services for people outside the mainstream of society, such as refugees and the homeless, face particular challenges in engaging and staying with their patients. Through necessity, such services set high standards in patient-centredness and the orchestration of care, which mainstream services would do well to follow.

12.1 WORKING WITH REFUGEES IN GENERAL PRACTICE

BECKY MACFARLANE

There is no stereotype of a refugee. They may be old or young, male or female, alone or with a spouse or a family group. They may be illiterate or have several university degrees, from a village or a megacity. They may have fled the indiscriminate destruction and chaos of war, been targeted as a member of a minority ethnic group or been subject to very personal intimidation, threats, detention and torture due to their political or religious activity or sexual orientation. Others seek humanitarian protection for themselves or a child from domestic violence or female genital mutilation. Some have been trafficked and seek protection after their escape. All face loneliness and fear, with separation from family and loss of home, job, status, possessions and all that is familiar.

It is common for them to face disbelief from authorities in the host country. This may lead to their being charged for health care provision which is free to the indigenous population, as is currently the case for refused asylum seekers in England (but not the rest of the United Kingdom) for secondary care and some community services. A fear of deportation to their country of origin may deter them from seeking health care or other help if they are not confident in the independence of the health care provider or other agency from the immigration authorities.

12.1.1 Understanding and negotiating the health system

All those seeking sanctuary in another country must negotiate a health care system, which is unfamiliar. It is important that they gain an understanding of how they can access medical help day or night, including the role of the GP as the usual first point of contact. This information may be provided by a statutory agency such as a specialist initial health assessment team or by a voluntary agency, which directs them to a local GP practice to register. Appointment systems may need to be explained as in many countries a person who is unwell simply goes to the hospital and waits to be seen.

12.1.2 Use of interpreters

Not being able to speak or read the language of the host country is a problem for many. Therefore, it is essential that an interpreting service is available. Gestures or the use of an online translation are not sufficient and can result in serious misunderstanding. Face-to-face interpreters are usually more effective, though in some situations phone interpreting is appropriate. Interpreters must be properly trained, preferably interpreting in the first person ('I have stomach pain' not 'She thinks she is pregnant'), and with a strict code of conduct including confidentiality and impartiality. Health care staff also benefit from training in how to work with interpreters. In emergencies, a family member or friend may be called upon to interpret; but this may hinder full disclosure of important issues, for example, where a parent does not want to give inappropriate information to a child.

12.1.3 Cultural understanding of health

People from different cultures understand and express health problems differently. Pain may indicate psychological distress, or illness may be regarded as a spiritual problem. There may be different beliefs about medicines. Some may have medicines sent over from their home country. Unfamiliarity with the concept of preventative treatment may cause poor compliance, for example, with an antihypertensive drug.

12.1.4 Initial health assessment

Initial assessment should include current problems. Trunk or limb injuries sustained during assault or torture or while fleeing may present with poorly healed fractures or other musculoskeletal damage. There may be head injuries requiring urgent investigation. A sensitive inquiry may elicit a history of rape of a woman or man and/or sexual activity on route requiring a sexual health screen. There may be an advanced pregnancy or immediate contraceptive needs. Questions should be asked to elicit symptoms of infection such as TB or parasites (cough, weight loss, night sweats, diarrhoea, abdominal pain). There may be symptoms of post-traumatic stress such as flashbacks, dissociation and hypervigilance.

A thorough past medical history is required including immunisation history, particularly in children (see http://apps.who.int/immunization_monitoring/globalsummary/schedules), which may be helpful. Medications may have different names. Congenital or developmental problems in children should be considered and may require further assessment.

It is helpful to ask about detention/imprisonment and torture by relating these to possible effects on health. There may be initial reluctance to disclose or discuss such experiences and a need for follow-up consultations to provide more time.

The basic examination of adults should include height, weight and blood pressure.

For adults, routine blood tests for HIV (for country prevalence >1%) and hepatitis B and C are recommended. HIV country prevalence data can be found at http://apps.who.int/gho/data/node.main.622?lang=en.

Routine full blood count is recommended to assess possible anaemia, particularly iron deficiency in women caused by menstruation, poor diet and helminth infestation such as hookworm. Eosinophilia may indicate parasitic infestation such as schistosomiasis.

Issues raised by initial assessment will lead to further investigation and referral as appropriate.

Conditions which may be more prevalent due to ethnicity, poor living conditions or lack of health care include type 2 diabetes in South Asians, fibroids in women of African origin, renal tract calculi, peptic ulcer, haemoglobinopathies, vitamin D deficiency/rickets, advanced inflammatory arthropathies, childhood eczema in Chinese, scabies and melasma in pale brown skin.

12.1.5 The realities of life for a refugee or asylum seeker

The complex asylum system and the circumstances that refugees face have a profound impact on health. Housing is provided on a no-choice basis, usually in deprived areas where there is empty council or private stock, which may be of poor quality. Cold, damp housing can exacerbate respiratory problems. Low levels of financial support and not being allowed to work during the processing of an application for asylum, and particularly withdrawal of all support and accommodation from those whose application is refused, can cause frustration, exhaustion and despair as well as vulnerability to exploitation such as illegal working for minimal pay or abusive sexual relationships. Some will experience immigration detention. The threat of detention or deportation causes great anxiety before and during the regular visit to the immigration reporting centre. There may be verbal or physical hostility from the local indigenous population, which increases fear and isolation.

Health may be improved, however, by good relationships both within and between communities. Refugee children, being relatively motivated and disciplined, can bring a boost to local schools. Adults may be able to contribute skills in community development. English classes and volunteering reduce isolation and improve future job prospects. Meeting with others of the same faith can bring a sense of belonging and shared identity.

12.1.6 The role of statutory and voluntary agencies

Third-sector agencies that support refugees are key in providing advice and practical support and assisting with orientation, integration and family reunion. These may be larger charities or smaller local groups.

The GP has an important role in emotional support, signposting, advocacy and building trust through continuity of care and confidentiality. The health visiting team can help to link families for mutual support or assist them to find local resources such as toddler groups or nursery provision. Social work referral can be made for those with care needs or a child in need.

Charities or specialist psychological trauma services supporting survivors of torture or other mistreatments may be able to provide formal documentation of evidence for the asylum application or appeal. The GP may be asked by a solicitor to provide a medical report confirming injuries or other health problems related to the reason for claiming asylum.

12.1.7 Conclusion

Refugees above all value a welcoming and kind manner and being listened to and believed. In this respect, they are no different to each one of us. To hear their experiences and to walk with them for part of their long journey is an inestimable privilege.

12.2 HOMELESS GENERAL PRACTICE

JOHN BUDD

Stewart presented with a painful and swollen left leg. He was worried because he was struggling to walk, making it difficult for him to get to his regular begging pitch.

He is in his early forties with a long history of mental health problems, having had multiple episodes of self-harm and overdoses and attracted the diagnosis of borderline personality disorder in his mid-20s. His drug and alcohol problems go back further into his teenage years, following on from an early childhood disrupted by family breakdown, neglect and being in care. Stewart has been homeless and in intermittent contact with our practice for the last 15 years, mainly attending for medical certificates.

Otherwise, he seems to have never quite been able to make use of our service, consistently declining any form of health care intervention. He is a frequent A+E attender, generally as a result of overdoses, injuries and intoxication. Over the last few years, he has been mainly sleeping rough, interspersed with periods in prison. Recently, concerns have been raised over Stewart's cognitive function and his ability to keep himself safe.

Clinically, he had a femoral deep vein thrombosis (DVT), as a result of groin injecting heroin. Liaising with an outreach worker, I tried several times to get Stewart seen at our local hospital, to get an ultrasound scan to confirm the diagnosis and start anti-coagulant treatment. However, on both occasions when

Stewart attended hospital, he refused to wait for the scan and refused hospital admission. So, I spoke once again to the outreach worker, who agreed to try and bring Stewart to one of my drop-in surgeries.

When Stewart arrived, we discussed how he seems to have struggled to make use of the hospital service. He was still in pain and so agreed to start an anti-coagulant treatment – without confirming the diagnosis – along with antibiotics. Stewart also reported feeling fed up with his 'lifestyle' of drug use and rough sleeping. I started him on methadone treatment, therefore, and his outreach worker managed to secure Stewart a room in a local supported homeless hostel. I was then able to introduce Stewart to one of my social work colleagues, in order to look at his wider care needs, in particular the management of his money.

Over the following weeks, Stewart managed to maintain his accommodation, complete his three-month course of anti-coagulation, stabilise on his methadone treatment and stop groin injecting heroin. He also agreed to link in with one of our mental health nurses, when he felt more able to look at some of his underlying psychological difficulties.

Stewart's history is not uncommon amongst patients attending homeless services. Many homeless patients suffer with the triple morbidity of physical and mental ill health, combined with substance use problems. Their health is further impacted by the experience of homelessness. The range and depth of these difficulties have led to this population group being described as 'multiply excluded homeless' (1) and suffering 'severe and multiple disadvantages'. This is characterised as being 'distinguishable from the other forms of social disadvantage because of the degree of stigma and dislocation from societal norms that these intersecting experiences represent as they push people to the edge of the mainstream' (2). The ensuing physical and mental health morbidity and mortality are catastrophic, with recent Scottish research finding a homeless population, with average age 42 and a burden of disease equivalent to that of people in their mid-80s in the general population (3).

Stewart's story also highlights some of the principles that underlie effective health care provision for people who are excluded and have multiple and complex problems: the importance of multidisciplinary and interagency working; open and flexible drop-in access, with the co-location of services operating under a harm reduction philosophy; the importance of assertive outreach for those that are not able or choose not to come to our health clinics.

And as a GP, I would emphasise the need for generalists at the heart of the service, to deal with the range and complexity of problems, supported by appropriate and accessible specialists when required. These principles clearly have relevance to mainstream practice, in that if we can get it right for those that struggle most to make use of our services, then we have the potential to get it right for all.

One core feature of health care services to vulnerable groups is of particular significance. We are increasingly aware that social dislocation and exclusion do not just affect people at random across society, but rather they have their roots in early life adversity and trauma, on a background of poverty – indeed the greatest risk factor for adult homelessness is childhood poverty (4). A growing body of research evidence is identifying the critical role of adverse childhood experiences (ACEs) in determining an individual's long-term health and social outcomes

(Section 11.3). The greater the number of ACEs and the greater their severity, such as physical or sexual abuse, the worse are the long-term outcomes for the child (5). A factor that has been shown to protect against the negative impact of adversity is the establishment of reliable, caring and trusting relationships (6).

The development of protective, trusting relationships also lies at the heart of providing effective health care to this patient group. The fostering of this type of relationship by services has come to be described as developing psychologically informed services or environments (PIE). Establishing trusting and potentially therapeutic relationships, with those for whom developing relationships is a major challenge, does not just involve clinicians. Rather, it needs to involve whole service design.

A psychologically informed approach will impact on the welcome patients receive at the front desk, the physical environment they encounter on entering the waiting room and how the service is structured, accessed and managed. It is a truly patient-centred model, taking as its starting point the difficulties that our patients, who have experienced early life trauma, have in establishing and making use of relationships.

This relational-based approach is perhaps the single most important feature of effective homeless health care services. Without this, the health care interventions that we offer are unlikely to be utilised effectively. In Stewart's case, our role as a GP practice has been to remain open and accessible, gently encouraging engagement and being ready to offer help when asked. With Stewart, it seems to have taken years for him to get to the point where he felt able to start making use of the health interventions that we have to offer. As a service, we need to be there when needed and in it for the long haul – the very essence of general practice.

REFERENCES

12.2 Homeless general practice

1. Fitzpatrick S, Bramley G, Johnsen S. 2012. Multiple Exclusion Homelessness in the UK: An overview of findings: Briefing Paper No. 1. Edinburgh, UK : Heriot-Watt University, 15 p.
2. Bramley G, Fitzpatrick S, Edwards J et al. 2015. *Hard Edges: Mapping Severe and Multiple Disadvantage in England*. The Lankelly Chase Foundation: London, UK.
3. Queen AB, Lowrie R, Richardson J, Williamson A. 2017. *BJGP Open*. doi:10.3399/bjgpopen17×100941.
4. Bramley G, Fitzpatrick S. 2017. Homelessness in the UK: Who is most at risk? *Housing Stud* 33:96–116. doi:10.1080/02673037.2017.1344957.
5. Felitti V, Anda R, Nordenberg D. 1998. Relationship of childhood abuse and household dysfunction to many of the leading causes of death in adults: The Adverse Childhood Experiences (ACE) study. *Am J Prev Med* 14:245–258.
6. Burley A. 2017. Choking up – relationships, multiple exclusion homelessness and psychologically informed environments. In *Homeless in Europe, Trauma and Homelessness*, pp. 8–10.

13

International perspectives

This section begins by describing the seven necessary components of health systems, as defined by the World Health Organization. Iona Heath then updates her *BMJ* article on "A general practitioner for every person in the world". This is followed by three international perspectives from Harry Wang and Stewart Mercer from China, Khairat Al Habbal and Mona Osman in Lebanon and Vincent Cubaka and Phil Cotton in Rwanda, describing the moves being made towards the development of primary care systems in these very different settings.

See also descriptions of general practice in Ireland (Section 6.2) and community practice in Ireland (Section 9.2), Australia (Section 9.3), the United States (Section 9.4) and Belgium (Section 9.5).

13.1 KEY COMPONENTS OF A WELL-FUNCTIONING HEALTH SYSTEM

Without strong policies and leadership, health systems do not spontaneously provide balanced response to the challenges they face, nor do they make the most efficient use of their resources. Health systems are subject to powerful forces and influences that often override rational policy making. These forces include disproportionate focus on specialist curative care, fragmentation in a multiplicity of competing programmes, projects and institutions, and the pervasive commercialization of health care delivery in poorly regulated systems. Keeping health systems on track requires a strong sense of direction and coherent investment in the various building blocks of the health system so as to provide the kind of services that produce results.

World Health Organization, 2010 (1)

For generalist clinical practice to be effective as a whole system, and not a scattered, heterogeneous and inefficient collection of small units, the following seven elements are required, all requiring central investment, support and coordination (1).

1. **Leadership** in primary care is needed not only at the top, determining the direction of travel and coordination of support services, but also at ground level, where often only local knowledge and experience can determine the best way forward.
2. **Governance procedures** are required so that the system, at every level, is accountable for the quality of care and use of public funds.
3. **Health information systems** allow progress to be reviewed, quality assessed, developments evaluated, practices compared and gaps identified.
4. **Health financing** reduces out-of-pocket expenditure on health care, the catastrophic financial effects of major illness and the ability to pay as a determinant of needs-based care.
5. **Human resources for health** comprise sufficient numbers of staff and efficient deployment of professional skills.
6. **Essential medical products and technologies** include the drugs and materials needed to deliver effective health care.
7. **Service delivery** to the whole population depends on effective, efficient and equitable systems of care.

In the WHO Report "Ten Years in Public Health, 2007–2017" (2), Nobel laureate Amartya Sen explains why universal health coverage is an "affordable dream" even for very poor countries. As he observes, many poor countries have shown that basic health care for all can be provided at a remarkably good level at very low cost if society, including its political and intellectual leadership, shows high-level commitment.

Sen refutes the common assumption that a poor country must first grow rich before it is able to meet the costs of health care for all. Health care is labour-intensive everywhere. A poor country with low wages may have less money to spend on health, but it also needs to spend less to provide these labour-intensive services.

Sen explains how universal health coverage provides greater equality, but also much larger overall health gains since it manages the most easily curable diseases and the prevention of easily avoidable diseases that are otherwise left out when systems rely on out-of-pocket payments (2).

Leading economists from 44 countries noted,

Health systems oriented towards universal health coverage, immensely valuable in their own right, produce an array of benefits: in times of crisis, they mitigate the effects of shocks on communities; in times of calm, they foster more cohesive societies and productive economies. (2)

13.2 A GENERAL PRACTITIONER FOR EVERY PERSON IN THE WORLD

IONA HEATH

*The year 2018 marks the 40th anniversary of the World Health Organization's Alma-Ata Declaration (1). This set the ambitious target of 'Health for All by the Year 2000' and was adopted in September 1978 at the International Conference on Primary HealthCare jointly sponsored by the WHO and UNICEF. The Declaration called for urgent action by all governments, health and development workers, and the world community to protect and promote the health of all the people of the world. The reasoning behind the target, laid out in Article X of the Declaration, was that 'an acceptable level of health for all the people of the world by the year 2000 can be attained through a fuller and better use of the world's resources, a considerable part of which is now spent on armaments and military conflicts.'

Tragically, since 1978, spending on war and armaments has continued unabated and is predicted to reach an obscene post-Cold War record of $1.67 trillion in 2018. Meanwhile, the Alma-Ata target came nowhere close to realisation and was replaced first by the United Nations' Millennium Development Goals for 2015, and now by the Sustainable Development Goals for 2030. It is frighteningly clear that this sequence is in danger of degenerating into an elaborate ritual, which provides the illusion of activity for the richer countries of the world while making very little difference to the realities of daily life for the world's poorest and most marginalised people.

It is no coincidence that Alma-Ata was the first international declaration to underline the central importance of primary health care:

> Governments have a responsibility for the health of their people which can be fulfilled only by the provision of adequate health and social measures. A main social target of governments, international organizations and the whole world community in the coming decades should be the attainment by all peoples of the world by the year 2000 of a level of health that will permit them to lead a socially and economically productive life. Primary health care is the key to attaining this target as part of development in the spirit of social justice.

Article VII provides a definition of primary health care and specifically refers to physicians as part of the health team at the local level. Yet, over the past 40 years, it has become increasingly obvious that part of the repeated failure of global health targets stems from the systematic neglect of the Alma-Ata vision of primary medical care as an essential component of primary health care.

* This is an updated version of an article previously published in the *BMJ* and included here with the Journal's permission. Heath I. A general practitioner for every person in the world. *BMJ* 2008;336:861. doi:10.1136/bmj.39548.435023.59.

In the rhetoric surrounding both the MDGs and the more recent SDGs, there has been much relevant discussion of the importance of universal health care coverage and the role of primary care in supporting that. However, the reference to the importance of primary care medicine has been minimal.

Unfortunately, following Alma-Ata, the commitment to comprehensive primary health care eroded rapidly. Just a year after the Alma-Ata Conference, an article in the *New England Journal of Medicine* opined:

> Until primary health care can be made available to all, services targeted to the few most important diseases may be the most effective means of improving the health of the greatest number of people. The crucial point is how to measure the effectiveness of medical interventions. (2)

This was the beginning of 'vertical programmes' focussing on single diseases such as HIV/AIDS, tuberculosis or malaria which recruit health care workers away from the 'horizontal' infrastructure of local health care. Vertical programs improve health care, but only for small groups of people with specific diseases. Some people receive good care; others remain untreated because there are no doctors, nurses, or medication available. To give just one example, the terrible Ebola epidemic of 2014–2015 fell resoundingly through the gaps between vertical programmes.

Yet, the tide had begun to turn again in 2008. Dr Halfdan Mahler had been the Director-General of WHO at the time of Alma-Ata and the WHO chose to mark the 30th anniversary of Alma-Ata by inviting him to address the World Health Assembly. He gave a wonderful short speech including this quotation from Milan Kundera:

> The struggle against human oppression is the struggle between memory and forgetfulness.

And this:

> When people are mere pawns in an economic and profit growth game, that game is mostly lost for the underprivileged.

> Let me postulate that if we could imagine a tabula rasa in health without having to deal with the constraints – tyranny if you wish – of the existing medical consumer industry, we would hardly go about dealing with health as we do now in the beginning of the 21st century.

Then in October 2008, the World Health Report was entitled "Primary Health Care – Now More Than Ever" and its contents offered a tantalising glimpse of the elusive possibility of letting memory triumph over forgetfulness (3). Yet, almost immediately forgetfulness was reasserting itself and this optimistic and impressive programme came under threat from the machinations of the big pharma–funded Non-Communicable Diseases Alliance, with the prospect of tackling health inequalities being reduced to the pursuit of risk factors for NCDs.

Underpinning all this, there seems to be an unspoken assumption that primary care physicians are a luxury that poor countries cannot afford and yet, in richer countries, they are the key to cost-effective health care systems and better health outcomes: surely just what is needed to achieve the health dimensions of any current and future Development Goals.

The painstaking work of Barbara Starfield and her team at Johns Hopkins University in Baltimore demonstrated that an increase in the number of primary care physicians for a given population is associated with a decrease in all-cause mortality. As the rising tide of overdiagnosis so clearly shows, contemporary medical care brings dangers as well as benefits and, when they are not undermined by ill-advised financial incentives, primary care physicians are trained to ensure that only those likely to benefit from specialist care are exposed to it. Beyond that, primary care physicians offer continuing relationships with individual patients and families which allow therapeutic interaction to extend over time in a context of trust and solidarity.

Poor people are no less aware of the skills of doctors than those who are more affluent, and many of the desperate parents whose children still die before the age of five in sub-Saharan Africa will incur crippling debt or sell vital livestock to see a private doctor if none is available to them through the public health care system. The poorest people in the poorest countries of the world are exposed to the most disease and therefore need commensurate access to properly trained doctors with broad diagnostic skills. Yet, they are the least likely to have access to trained general practitioners or family doctors. Only when every person in the world has a general practitioner will we know that those in power are serious about Health for All.

13.3 PERSPECTIVE FROM CHINA

HARRY HAO-XIANG WANG AND STEWART W. MERCER

China is the world's most populous country and has been shaping its primary care provision during the past several decades (1). At the moment, national policy is that primary care facilities are being established as the backbone of the entire health system to broaden equitable access to primary care and reduce the spread of chronic conditions and multimorbidity. In rural areas, township health centres (THCs) and village clinics are the core primary care providers. In urban areas, primary care is mainly provided by community health centres and subordinate stations (CHCs). Primary care is being characterised by the service provision of a six-in-one care package integrating health prevention, protection, treatment, rehabilitation, education and family planning (2).

Similar to the UK and other countries worldwide, China faces multifactorial challenges including rapid ageing, unhealthy lifestyles, psychosocial factors, environmental hazards and many other emerging risk factors. A major characteristic in China is that the health system, dominated by secondary care, is hospital-centric and volume-driven. In the absence of gatekeeping, people often bypass primary care facilities and go straight to hospitals. Repeated clinical examinations and multiple medication prescriptions due to episode-based visits to different hospitals are common, particularly among those with multimorbidity (3).

Fragmentation in care, associated with specialism, in conjunction with people's long-existing bias against generalism, often leads to the escalation of out-of-pocket payments. In contrast with public perceptions, research has shown that generalists at CHCs provide better primary care, compared with specialists at outpatient departments in hospitals (4). Responding to the rising treatment burden and the challenge of keeping the population well and living outside hospitals for as long as possible through effective primary care approach remains a particular priority.

Safe, effective, convenient and affordable basic care are the expected deliverables of clinical generalism in the primary care setting, where both curative and preventive care services are being delivered.

Essential medical care in China covers

- Disease treatment of major and common infectious diseases, endemic diseases, as well as parasitic diseases
- Diagnosis and treatment of common health problems
- Basic acute care
- Referral services coordinated with hospitals

Essential public health care covers

- Establishment of health profiles and medical records
- Provision of health education
- Disease prevention and vaccination
- Health management for targeted high-risk populations, including children (aged 0–6 years), the elderly (aged 65 years and above), women (pregnancy and postpartum care), and patients with hypertension, type 2 diabetes, tuberculosis or serious mental illness
- Health management with traditional Chinese medicine
- Reporting of and responding to infectious diseases and public health emergencies
- Sanitation control and monitoring

Increasing access to primary care requires substantial general practice capacity building to tackle the complexity of health problems encountered. Nevertheless, due to the absence of undergraduate-level education in GP, a majority of GP physicians working in primary care receive inadequate education and training. The Primary Care Assessment Tool showed a suboptimal level of the community orientation attribute of China's primary care, when compared with first contact, continuity, coordination and comprehensiveness from patients' experiences (5).

The identified gap in service delivery requires GP physicians to pay more attention to patients' personal beliefs, health attitudes and lifestyle changes rather than disease treatment. This highlights the need for clinical generalism with the capability of improving population health outcomes in the presence of a broad spectrum of health risk factors.

In response to the Healthy China 2030 agenda, the 'family doctor team' is an emerging primary care model characterised by cohesive health management service provision that embraces family centred continuous care as opposed to episodic care. The concept is based on the complexity of patients' care, including the provision of health management starting with perspectives that take into account the wider determinants of health. On top of routine curative care such as the diagnosis and treatment of common disorders, frequently occurring diseases, and non-serious acute conditions or injuries, the service package also covers a wide range of preventive care including health assessment, health interventions with follow-ups, health advice, and when necessary, home visits.

The number of staff within a doctor team in a primary care facility is determined by the number of GP physicians. A typical family doctor team is comprised of one GP physician and others including nurses, public health doctors, and if possible, pharmacists, psychology consultants and social workers. Having holistic care provided and managed by an interdisciplinary team instead of by a GP physician alone takes into account both the physician shortage and the need for more complex patient care. A contract on care delivery is signed between the GP and the individual residents at registration. The team as a whole assumes responsibility for the health of registered individuals and those who live together in the same family, whilst service users are encouraged to seek care initially from the family doctor team for non-urgent problems.

The adoption of family doctor teams has many implications. The long-existing fee-for-service payment methods used since the 1990s in China tend to reward high-volume services for disease treatment where perverse incentives from prescribing examinations and drugs aggravated many problems. With a contract co-signed between GP physicians and individual patients, the GP-led family doctor team is given responsibility for a panel of registered people including healthy individuals, at-risk individuals and patients already suffering from diseases who commit to care by the team.

Thus, the GP physician has a leadership role, leading the whole team to their best endeavours in a generalist approach following primary care principles to deliver both patient-centred and population-oriented services. Since primary care facilities are encouraged to develop family doctor teams, professionals from a variety of disciplines sharing unique perspectives can thus expand the scope of clinical generalism and lighten the GP physician's load.

With the implementation of the family doctor team approach, there is a call for changing the way in which primary care providers, particularly GP physicians, are educated and trained so that clinical generalism lies at the heart of care delivery in response to population health needs, which are diverse and complex. To respond to this challenge, GP physicians are required to have proper knowledge, adequate skills, professional values and positive attitudes to the delivery of collaborative primary care. Enhancing people's confidence in clinical generalism and attracting highly qualified GP physicians is important. Factors strongly associated with entering primary care practice include a well-formulated curriculum with exposure to the community, positive clinical and public health experiences as part of education and training and optimistic attitudes toward generalism.

A nationwide '5 + 3' mechanism for GP physicians has been adopted across China recently. This starts with five years of undergraduate-level clinical education (including traditional Chinese medicine) followed by three years of structured postgraduate education with a masters degree. A typical GP education and training structure are underpinned by theoretical learning, field practice based on clinical rotation, and community-based practice with early exposure to the complexity of care. Theoretical teaching includes conventional lecture-based learning and problem-based learning, whilst practical teaching in general practice takes place at a wide range of primary care facilities where GP trainees can experience the clinical diversity of both prevention and treatment activities for chronic diseases and multimorbidity in daily practice.

The increasing needs for preventive care, regular health examinations and follow-up care have been surged in the community where generalism can be translated from theory into action within the family doctor team. This is the future direction for GPs working in primary care in China. At the moment, prospective studies are being performed to assess the long-term effect of primary care generalism on population health.

13.4 PERSPECTIVE FROM LEBANON

KHAIRAT AL HABBAL AND MONA OSMAN

Lebanon is a middle-income country with a population of around 5.8 million (1) including Syrian and Palestinian refugees. The country has passed through several crises including a protracted civil war (1975–1990) that halted the growth of the public health care system (2). Prior to the war, the government enacted legislation that gave medical graduates the option of practising in rural areas for two years as a substitute for pursuing further specialty training. The law was intended to increase primary health care coverage in rural areas but unfortunately led to an increase in the number of specialists (2). The war then exacerbated this situation by destroying many of the public health care facilities. The private sector filled the gap and developed curative rather than primary health care services which increased the cost of the health bill. This posed and still poses a problem since less than half of the population has health insurance in the form of a private insurance package or one of six employment-based social insurance funds. Others are covered by the Ministry of Public Health (MoPH) for secondary and tertiary care, thus necessitating out-of-pocket payments for primary health care services (3).

The health care system in Lebanon is based on private public partnership with a high percentage of specialists. Patients can access specialists directly and freely; there is an absence of gate-keeping. Only 30% of registered doctors are in general medicine or family medicine (2). General practitioners (GPs) differ from family physicians (FP) in Lebanon in that GPs do not pursue any vocational or specialty training after graduating from medical school, whereas family doctors complete a residency program of three to four years. A recent law issued in 2014 (law number 271), from which existing GPs are exempted, prohibits the practice of medicine in the country without having at least three years of specialty training after medical school.

The first family medicine residency program in the country and the region started in 1979 (4). Four more residency programs are currently available of which three were launched within the last five years including one in the only public university in the country. The number of family medicine graduates per year is estimated to be around 18 to 20. There are currently around 120 practicing family physicians in the country, with less than 1 doctor per 37,000 population, not including refugees.

Given this context, what is the situation of clinical generalism and is there a role for it in Lebanon?

From a field perspective, family practice involves the medicine of the extremes. People of lower socioeconomic status (SES) cannot afford health care except at primary health care centers (PHCCs) where they are seen by GPs or FPs. This gives the impression that FPs are the doctors of the poor. It stems from the historical background of the first fifteen years post-independence (1943–1958) when the government built a network of care for the underprivileged and asked for evidence of financial need before admitting them for care. The resulting stigma associated with use of public services remains an issue to this day (2). On the other end of the spectrum, there is a proportion of the population with high SES who have lived abroad in countries where a family physician is the gatekeeper to care. They may seek an FP's opinion in his/her private clinic. The remainder of the population is often seen by specialists in their private clinics or in PHCCs.

A survey conducted among practising FPs (5) revealed that they remain enthusiastic about their profession despite many challenges. Many opt to have a stable income, rather than just relying on income from consultations, thus taking on more administrative or hospital-based work. They also maintain a good relationship with specialists.

In past years, more work has been done to strengthen family practice and integrate it in primary health care services. The World Health Organization Eastern Mediterranean Region Office (WHO-EMRO) adopted the concept of family practice for the effective and efficient delivery of primary health care services (6). The Syrian Refugee crisis added further burden to the Lebanese health care system, necessitating the need for stronger primary health care services to address the needs of both the citizens and refugees (7). This has led to an increased number of residency programs and the development of bridging programs for GPs in collaboration with WHO as well as developing new programs at the level of the MoPH that aim to strengthen primary health care services, such as the accreditation of primary health care centers, developing health packages (based on preventive services) as a step towards universal health coverage and other programs that aim to integrate primary care at the community level.

More work still needs to be done at different levels to strengthen the role of family physicians in general. This includes, for example, mandating to have FPs as the first contact before passing to other levels of care, better career orientation for medical students highlighting the importance of family practice and raising awareness among the public of the crucial role of family physicians and generalism in general.

13.5 PERSPECTIVE FROM SUB-SAHARAN AFRICA

VINCENT CUBAKA AND PHIL COTTON

It is challenging to describe primary health care in sub-Saharan Africa as it varies across countries and within countries. There are differences but also similarities in terms of context, health needs and health policy that determine the framework of primary health care, its relationship with the rest of the health system, the type of health care provider and their scope of practice.

Africa is currently the second most populous continent in the world with over a billion people (1). Most sub-Saharan African countries are low-income countries. There are gross inequalities and disparities in social economic status, health status and health care within and between countries as well as between sub-Saharan Africa and the rest of the world (2). The majority of the population is rural, poor and with low literacy levels. This often determines the epidemiological picture but not necessarily the priorities of national health systems (3).

Most national health systems are pyramidal with three common levels consisting of tertiary care hospitals at the top, led by specialists, followed by secondary care – provincial, district, or county hospitals, often led by medical officers without any postgraduate education, and at the bottom primary health care facilities – clinics, health centres, dispensaries, health posts, and so on. These primary health care facilities are often led by nurses or mid-level cadres (non-physician clinicians). They generally provide curative and preventive health services including ambulatory care, maternity care, antenatal care, child immunization, family planning, HIV/AIDS care, TB care, and so on. In general, there are few or no medical doctors in primary health care in African countries.

Primary health care in the majority of sub-Saharan Africa countries is typically characterised by:

- Being part of poorly organised and managed (i.e. weak) national health systems, as revealed by the recent Ebola outbreak in Guinea, Liberia and Sierra Leone (4)
- A context that promotes and relies on specialty care in city-based hospitals (5)
- An 'inverse primary health care law', whereby the limited resources, including the shortage of health workforce, contrast with a heavy burden of the disease and health needs (6,7). The majority of resources go to secondary and tertiary care hospitals, caring for a small portion of the population (5).
- Vertical, disease-oriented and donor-driven programs that prioritise infectious diseases (HIV, malaria, tuberculosis), maternal and child health and more recently, non-communicable diseases, rationalised by an increasing burden of communicable and non-communicable diseases and high child and maternal mortality (8).

Primary health care is increasingly recognised as the backbone of health systems. Still, in several sub-Saharan African countries, it is not used to its full potential and is sometimes undervalued, being generally and erroneously considered cheap and, therefore, of poor quality (9). People who can afford it bypass primary health care facilities and head straight to ambulatory care provided by doctors in hospitals, with the assumption that care will be better. In addition, the scarce primary health care workforce is poorly prepared, supported and motivated, and often overburdened, leading to high staff turnover and out-migration (7).

These problems are exacerbated in remote and deprived areas and constitute a recipe for poor health outcomes as reflected in health indicators from the region (10). Furthermore, as with health systems generally, primary health care action is often dispersed among different actors, including public institutions, NGOs, the private health sector, faith-based institutions and traditional healers, often with poor coordination. This situation leads to inequitable and unsustainable access to health services with a mixed impact. For example, in Nigeria, the inadequacy of the public health system has given an increasingly important role to the private health sector as well as to traditional and spiritual healers (11).

Despite all the above issues, during the last decade, sub-Saharan African countries have made progress in improving the health of populations by strengthening their health systems and endorsing the primary health care approach, with the help of partners like WHO (1). For instance, Rwanda has improved several national health indicators thanks to strong political will, a decentralization policy, strong community-based health assurance, the expansion of primary health care facilities (health centres) and a network of community health workers (12). Much still needs to be done, including training and deployment of more community-oriented doctors to improve clinical generalism and to support district and primary health care teams.

During recent decades, several African countries have launched postgraduate family medicine programs with the aim of training community-oriented doctors who will strengthen primary health care. These countries include South Africa (often seen as the role model), Ghana, Nigeria, Lesotho, Mozambique, Tanzania, Kenya, Uganda, Sudan, Democratic Republic of Congo, Rwanda, Zambia and most recently Botswana, Mali, Somaliland, Malawi and Ethiopia and soon Zimbabwe. These initiatives are supported by networks and organizations like WONCA (World Organization of Family Doctors), PRIMAFAMED (Primary HealthCare and Family Medicine Education) and the Besrour Centre (of the College of Family Physician of Canada) (13,14). While the potential role and impact of family physicians in African countries are still being explored, we believe it represents the way forward to clinical generalism and strong primary health care in sub-Saharan Africa (15). Indeed, there is evidence that primary health care backed by community-oriented and socially accountable doctors can help to improve and maintain the health of communities (16).

In Africa, with few exceptions, medical education focuses on clinical readiness rather than stewardship roles (17). Health managers and policymakers may or may not have a clinical background. While the role of family medicine in Africa is developing, we believe that with curricula that also focus on stewardship skills, family medicine can help to bridge the gap between practice and policy. Indeed, family doctors who play a leadership role in multidisciplinary health teams may help strengthen primary health care more effectively and have a much greater impact on the health system. This stewardship responsibility of African family doctors needs to be further explored and eventually expanded.

REFERENCES

13.1 Key components of a well-functioning health system

1. World Health Organization. Everybody's business: Strengthening health systems to improve health outcomes: WHO's framework for action. WHO, 2007. www.who.int/healthsystems/strategy/everybodys_business.pdf
2. World Health Organization. Ten years of Public Health 2007–2017: Report by Dr Margaret Chan, Director-General, World Health Organization 2017. Available from http://www.who.int/publications/10-year-review/universal-coverage/en/index5.html.

13.2 A general practitioner for every person in the world

1. World Health Organization. Declaration of Alma-Ata. World Health Organization, 1978
2. Walsh JA, Warren KS. Selective primary health care: An interim strategy for disease control in developing countries. *N Engl J Med* 1979;301:967–974.
3. World Health Report 008. Primary health care now more than ever. World Health Organization, Geneva, Switzerland, 2008.

13.3 Perspective from China

1. Wang HHX, Wang JJ. Chapter 40 developing primary care in China. In: Griffiths SM, Tang JL, Yeoh EK, Eds. *Routledge Handbook of Global Public Health in Asia*. Taylor & Francis Group, London, UK, 2014 April, pp. 584–600.
2. Wang HHX, Wang JJ, Wong SYS, Wong MCS, Mercer SW, Griffiths SM. The development of urban community health centres for strengthening primary care in China: A systematic literature review. *Br Med Bull* 2015;116:139–153.
3. Wang HHX, Wang JJ, Wong SYS, Wong MCS, Li FJ, Wang PX, Zhou ZH, Zhu CY, Griffiths SM, Mercer SW. Epidemiology of multimorbidity in China and implications for the healthcare system: cross-sectional survey among 162,464 community household residents in southern China. *BMC Med* 2014;12:188, 12 pages.
4. Wang HHX, Wong SYS, Wong MCS, Wei XL, Wang JJ, Li DKT, Tang JL, Gao GY, Griffiths SM. Patients' experiences in different models of community health centers in southern China. *Ann Fam Med* 2013;11:517–526.
5. Wang HHX, Wong SYS, Wong MCS, Wang JJ, Wei XL, Li DKT, Tang JL, Griffiths SM. Attributes of primary care in community health centres in China and implications for equitable care: A cross-sectional measurement of patients' experiences. *QJM-An Int J Med* 2015;108:549–560.

13.4 Perspective from Lebanon

1. World Health Organization. Countries. Lebanon. http://www.who.int/countries/lbn/en/ (Accessed on February 25, 2018).
2. Kronfol N. Older population and health system: A profile of Lebanon, 2008. Available from http://www.who.int/ageing/projects/intra/phase_one/alc_intra1_cp_lebanon.pdf (accessed on 27 February 2018).
3. World Health Organization. Country Cooperation Strategy for WHO and Lebanon 2010–2015. Available from http://www.who.int/country-cooperation/publications/en/ (accessed 25 February 2018).
4. Arya N, Gibson C, Ponka D, Haq C, Hansel S, Dahlman B, Rouleau K. Family medicine around the world: Overview by region. *Can Fam Physician* 2017;63:436–441.
5. Helou M, Rizk GA. State of family medicine practice in Lebanon. *J Family Med Prim Care* 2016;5:51–55.
6. World Health Organization–Regional Office for the Eastern Mediterranean. Conceptual and strategic approach to family practice: Towards universal health coverage through family practice in the Eastern Mediterranean Region, 2014. Available from http://applications.emro.who.int/dsaf/EMROPUB_2014_EN_1783.pdf.
7. Ammar W, Kdouh O, Hammoud R, Hamadeh R, Harb H, Ammar Z, Atun R, Christiani D, Zalloua PA. Health system resilience: Lebanon and the Syrian refugee crisis. *J Glob Health* 2016;6:020704. doi:10.7189/jogh.06.020704.

13.5 Perspective from sub-Saharan Africa

1. World Health Organization. Regional Office for Africa. The health of the people: What works – The African Regional Health Report 2014 [Internet]. World Health Organization, Geneva, Switzerland, 2014. Available from http://apps.who.int/iris/bitstream/handle/10665/137377/9789290232612.pdf?sequence=4.
2. Mash RB, Reid S. Statement of consensus on family medicine in Africa. *Afr J Prim Health Care Fam Med* 2010;2:1–4.
3. World Health Organization. Regional Office for Africa. The health of the people: The African regional health report/World Health Organization, Regional Office for Africa [Internet]. Africa WHORO for, editor. Brazzaville, Republic of Congo: World Health Organization, Regional Office for Africa; 2006. 170 p. Available from http://www.who.int/bulletin/africanhealth/en/index.html.
4. Boozary AS, Farmer PE, Jha AK. The Ebola outbreak, fragile health systems, and quality as a cure. *JAMA* 2014;1859–1860.
5. De Maeseneer J, Flinkenflögel M. Primary health care in Africa: Do family physicians fit in? *Br J Gen Pract* 2010;286–292.

6. Willcox ML, Peersman W, Daou P, Diakité C, Bajunirwe F, Mubangizi V, et al. Human resources for primary health care in sub-Saharan Africa: Progress or stagnation? *Hum Resour Health* 2015;13(1). doi:10.1186/s12960-015-0073-8.

7. Moosa S, Wojczewski S, Hoffman K, Poppe A, Nkomazana O, Peersman W et al. Why there is an inverse primary-care law in Africa. *Lancet Glob Health* 2013;1(6):e332–e333.

8. De Maeseneer J. Primary health care in Africa: Now more than ever! *Afr J Prim Health Care Fam Med* 2009;1(1):1–3.

9. World Health Organization, WHO. Primary health care now more than ever. *World Heal Rep* 2008;996(10):148. Available from http://www.who.int/whr/2008/whr08_en.pdf.

10. Bangdiwala S, Fonn S, Okoye O, Tollman S. Workforce resources for health in developing countries. *Public Health Rev* 2010;32:296–318.

11. Gyuse AN, Ayuk AE, Okeke MC. Facilitators and barriers to effective primary health care in Nigeria. *African J Prim Heal Care Fam Med* 201821;10(1):1641. Available from http://www.ncbi.nlm.nih.gov/pmc/articles/PMC5843931/.

12. Sayinzoga F, Bijlmakers L. Drivers of improved health sector performance in Rwanda: A qualitative view from within. *BMC Health Serv Res* 2016;16(1):123.

13. Arya N, Gibson C, Ponka D, Haq C, Hansel S, Dahlman B et al. Family medicine around the world: Overview by region: The Besrour papers: A series on the state of family medicine in the world. *Can Fam Physician* 2017;436–441.

14. Ray SC, Masuka N. Facilitators and barriers to effective primary health care in Zimbabwe. *African J Prim Heal Care Fam Med* 2017;9(1):1639.

15. Mash R, Downing R, Moosa S, De Maeseneer J. Exploring the key principles of Family Medicine in sub-Saharan Africa: International Delphi consensus process. *South African Fam Pract* 2008;50(3):60–65.

16. Kidd MR. *The Contribution of Family Medicine to Improving Health Systems: A Guidebook from the World Organization of Family Doctors*, 2nd edition. International Journal of Health Care Quality Assurance, Singapore, 2013. Available from http://www.globalfamilydoctor.com/InternationalIssues/WONCAGuidebook.aspx%5Cnhttp://www.emeraldinsight.com/doi/10.1108/IJHCQA.06226gaa.014.

17. Eyal N, Cancedda C, Kyamanywa P, Hurst SA. Non-physician clinicians in sub-Saharan Africa and the evolving role of physicians. *Int J Heal Policy Manag* 2015;5(3):149–153.

14

Working to produce evidence of change

Monsieur Diderot, I have listened with the greatest pleasure to all the inspirations of your brilliant mind. But all your grand principles, which I understand very well, would do splendidly in books and very badly in practice. In your plans for reform, you are forgetting the difference between our two positions: you work only on paper which accepts anything, is smooth and flexible and offers no obstacles either to your imagination or your pen, while I, poor empress, work on human skin, which is far more sensitive and touchy.

Catherine the Great to the French Enlightenment Philosopher Denis Diderot (1)

Some types of research are easy to carry out on a controlled, sometimes industrial, scale, either within laboratories or networks of specialised clinics. Research in the community, involving people going about their ordinary lives whether at work or at home, presents a very different challenge.

Every study is a social construction in which the necessary relationships and behaviours are established in order to create the temporary moment when a clear answer is obtained for a clear research question.

The skills to achieve this are seldom taught in courses on research methods that concentrate on research design and statistical analysis. These aspects of research are important, but research teams in the community also need to be streetwise.

The UK Medical Research Council Epidemiology Research Unit, led by Professor Archie Cochrane, pioneered high-population response rates in the 1950s with a series of epidemiological studies in the South Wales mining valleys, often achieving participation rates of 90–95% (2). Famously, when the professor asked his team for the addresses of people who had not participated so that he could visit them himself and offer a lift to the research clinic in his Daimler, he recruited not a single extra person. His research team of local people, who knew their communities well, had already exhausted what their communities could deliver.

I had the good fortune to work with a very streetwise research team led by Mary Hart, in Julian Tudor Hart's general practice at Glyncorrwg in South Wales in the early 1980s. Both had worked previously in the MRC Epidemiology Unit. A preliminary study assessed daily salt intake in 90% of 116 participants based on the collection of seven consecutive 24-hour urine collections – a huge imposition on the day-to-day lives of men and women at work, at home and in their leisure time (3).

The main intervention studies that followed involved firstly 18 patients with mild hypertension (4) and then 66 young adults with and without a family history of high blood pressure in 10 weeks of dietary salt restriction, reducing intakes from 8 to 3 grams per day (the level of South Seas islanders) while taking part in a randomised double-blind controlled trial of tablets containing either sodium chloride or placebo (5). As most salt in the diet is added during food processing, participants were provided with low-sodium bread and a range of other low-sodium foodstuffs.

Such a study, with its participation and achievement rates, could perhaps only take place in a general practice setting but, even so, it was unprecedented and is unlikely ever to be repeated. With this personal experience, I was in no doubt that a book about the exceptional potential of general practice should include contributions on how to engage with general practices for research and evaluation.

Bridie Fitzpatrick is Scotland's leading exponent of delivering large and complex research studies, including general practices serving very deprived areas. In her contribution below, she describes her rules of engagement with reference to the Care Plus Study (Section 3.4).

The practical research challenge is usually to deliver a pre-specified protocol in a particular setting. The contrast in service development work is that the nature of the changes to be made are often unknowable at the outset and only emerge slowly by trial and error as changes are customised to the local setting. Jamie Sinclair describes working in this way in a project involving the embedding of a financial advisor in two Deep End general practices.

14.1 RULES OF ENGAGEMENT

BRIDIE FITZPATRICK

This section draws on three and a half decades of experience of conducting a wide range of research projects from large epidemiological studies to small trials of complex interventions. Regardless of their focus, all have relied on obtaining data from health care settings, most recently general practice.

In many ways, carrying out a research project is like executing a military campaign. Both have an overall aim, specific objectives, a plan of action, desired outcomes and, but not always, an exit plan. However, success in research relies on engagement and reconciliation of interests rather than force.

Projects, by definition, are extraordinary to routine practice and consequently require people to change the way they work by doing additional activities and/or make adjustments to their usual activities. Thus, success in research relies on strategies employed and actions taken to recognise and overcome potential conflicts of interest, ideally before they arise, and to engage all the relevant parties throughout all phases of the project, from translating the study protocol into a detailed operational plan, through execution of that plan to cessation of activity. The rules described here may also apply to testing new ways of working.

1. **Know your target**: Potential patient research participants are likely to have gatekeepers whose participation and/or support is required e.g. GP practice staff. It is important to recognise that the primary concern of staff is their current response to patient need. Consequently, it is important to understand what motivates the gatekeepers and research participants to engage in research as well as the barriers to overcome.
2. **Invest in reconnaissance and establish collaborators**: Similar practice settings can be operationally very different. Spending time on reconnaissance can provide useful insights e.g. is there someone in the organisation who can effectively influence the pass of information to and from the gatekeeper of the research participants – i.e. a 'gatekeeper' of the gatekeeper. Collaborators include all research participants as well as the gatekeepers to them and other potential sources of data. It involves fostering joint ownership whereby ambitions for the project's success are shared.
3. **Maintain visibility**: This is chiefly concerned with creating and maintaining interest in the research study. Key members of the research team should meet their collaborators in person at the outset of the study (to become a 'kent' face) and maintain a visible presence throughout its duration.
4. **Produce a realistic detailed operational plan**: At the outset, think through all the steps required to achieve the project's overall aim and be realistic in terms of available resources (financial, human and time). This involves identifying all the individual components required, putting them together and recognising the maintenance measures needed to keep the project running efficiently and effectively.
5. **Strategically appoint a research team**: The person responsible for managing the research must understand the work involved in all activities in the operational plan and the skill sets required by the individuals taking part. Key considerations in appointing staff include their ability to demonstrate compliance with professional standards and adherence to standardised operational procedures; attention to detail and good record keeping; flexibility and tenacity in pursuit of objectives; and excellent interpersonal skills.
6. **Establish clear lines of communication**: Lines of the communication for the research team should be detailed for each of the study processes in a standardised operating procedure. Lines of communication for research collaborators should be prominent in all the study information materials and reiterated in contacts with the research team.

7. **Establishing systems for monitoring progress and implementing contingency plans**: Data capturing systems are required to assess actual achievements against planned achievements such as the implementation of the planned intervention as well as recruitment and retention rates. This allows discrepancies to be reviewed and when necessary the implementation of contingency plans.

8. **Maintain morale and lead by example**: Attention to esprit de corps extends beyond the research team, includes all research collaborators and is chiefly concerned with maintaining everyone's belief in the importance of the project. It involves ensuring that everyone is properly equipped and rewarded. The person with overall responsibility should lead by example and be prepared to work alongside the research team, particularly during labour-intensive periods or in the face of difficulty.

9. **Have an exit plan**: This involves ensuring that everyone is abreast with project timelines, progress and results. The benefits of this are likely to extend beyond the lifetime of the project and may lead to participation in future research.

The success of the CARE Plus Study was described in Section 3.4 and is used below to illustrate some of the above rules in action.

Four participating general practices were randomised to deliver the intervention whilst the other four provided usual care. For all practices, data were collected from several sources including self-completed questionnaires from participating staff and patients (at three separate time points); CARE and Enablement questionnaires (1,2) data from a sample of patients before and after routine consultations on two occasions; and data on service use by the participating patients (at one time point). Additionally, intervention practitioners completed a bespoke record for each CARE Plus consultation and patients completed a questionnaire after their first CARE Plus consultation. These allowed assessments of the extent to which the study intervention was implemented as intended.

Thus, participation in the study involved significant additional work for all practices. Numerous strategies were developed to understand, engage and maintain the interest and support of key members of practice teams, particularly those who were disappointed that their practice had not been randomised to deliver the intervention. These involved key members of the research team, including the study administrator, meeting practice staff to set up the study in a manner that would cause least disruption to their usual activities. Interest and collaboration were maintained by visiting the GP practices in person either formally before each round of data collection or informally with biscuits or sweets as small tokens of appreciation.

These visits also provided the opportunity to discuss how the study impacted on the practices' routine activities and vice versa, and to ensure that they were being adequately remunerated for additional work. When necessary, facilitation measures were put in place. For example, collection of the CARE and Enablement questionnaire data was coordinated so that they could feed into GP revalidation activities.

Patient participant outcome measures were obtained using a 14-page questionnaire. At the onset of the study, the questionnaire was administered by a member of the research team in a face-to-face meeting with each patient. Whilst resource intensive, this served a number of purposes including the opportunity to personalise the study, familiarise participants with the study questionnaire and achieve a mutual understanding of what participation would entail.

This tactic paid dividends in achieving high retention rates at two follow-up periods and reducing the need for face-to-face meetings (34% at 6 months and 22% at 12 months). The other questionnaires were administered either by a researcher in a telephone interview (9% at 6 months and 13% at 12 months) or were completed and returned by the patient by mail in a prepaid, pre-addressed envelope (57% at 6 months and 65% at 12 months). Patients' travel expenses were reimbursed and they were given a £5 gift voucher as a token of appreciation each time they completed a questionnaire.

The study logo helped brand and maintain the visibility of the study, being used on all written correspondence, including seasonal greetings cards and progress reports between periods of data collection.

In addition to the work associated with mailing and acknowledging receipt of study questionnaires, each round of data collection entailed substantial email and telephone correspondence. For example, the total number of contact attempts (successful and unsuccessful) to patient participants was 2,025 at the start of the study (patient mean 8.96), 835 at 6 months follow-up (patient mean 5.68), and 1,056 at 12 months follow-up (patient mean 7.14). This was a team effort involving some out-of-hours work. Formal and informal arrangements to maintain morale included regular team meetings, meals out and board games/jigsaws in the team's breakout area in the office.

14.2 THE DEEP END ADVICE WORKER PROJECT

JAMIE SINCLAIR

14.2.1 Overview

Building on the well-established model of co-locating social and economic support in general practice (GP) settings, the Deep End Advice Worker Project developed and tested approaches to delivering advice from two general practices in Parkhead, Glasgow (1). Through the delivery of finance, debt, social security and housing advice from a trusted setting, the project aimed to improve social and economic outcomes for patients in the practice. It also sought to reduce the time medical staff spent on non-clinical issues.

14.2.2 Deep End general practices

The project involved two general practices in Parkhead, Glasgow. Recent Scottish Index of Multiple Deprivation (SIMD) data positions Parkhead as one of the most deprived areas in Scotland. The practices are classed as the fifth and eleventh most deprived GP practices in Scotland (out of 951 practices) and support 3,192 and 4,711 patients, respectively.

14.2.3 Origin of the project

The Wheatley Housing Group in Glasgow had spare end of year money and wished to try placing financial advice in general practices serving deprived areas. They contacted the Deep End group and were put in touch with two suitable practices which were not involved in any other Deep End Projects. The Greater Easterhouse Money Advice Project (GEMAP) provided an advice worker. The Glasgow Centre for Population Health (GCPH) offered evaluation, attaching a colleague from Building Connections. Health improvement colleagues from Greater Glasgow and Clyde NHS coordinated planning meetings which, after a poorly attended first meeting at the GCPH, were all held at Parkhead Health Centre.

14.2.4 Outcomes

Between December 2015 and May 2017, the Deep End Advice Worker Project secured the following outcomes:

- 276 referrals
- 235 (85%) had never previously accessed GEMAP's services
- 165 people engaged with the service once referred (65% engagement rate)
- £848,001 worth of financial gain was secured through income maximisation work
- £155,766 worth of debt was identified and managed

The median financial gain for patients accessing advice was £6,967 per person, per annum. Considering that 128 (78%) of people accessing the service were living on household incomes of less than £15,000 per annum, the amount of financial gain is significant. The project generated substantial additional income for people through ensuring they received the social security payments to which they were entitled.

14.2.5 Embedding advice workers in general practice settings

The project did not involve an advice worker parachuting into the practices to deliver a separate service. Instead, we attempted to embed the advice worker into the everyday work of the two general practices. In this way, partner organisations sought to normalise the availability of expert social and economic advice and the advice worker's presence in the practices to the extent that referrals to the service were viewed in the same way as referrals to other NHS health services.

Several steps were taken to help embed the advice worker in the practice team. For example, first name introductions to all practice staff; the provision of a consultation room to deliver advice; and access to information from medical records when required.

The advice worker attended for half a day per week in each practice. GPs and frontline staff made referrals through a secure online system. Referrals were explicitly framed as an additional form of support, not a replacement for a GP appointment. First meetings took place in a consultation room in the patient's practice. Home visits were also available. With the consent of the patient, the advice worker was able to access information from medical records to inform the preparation of social security applications.

14.2.6 Medical records

Access to information in medical records (with written patient consent) provided the advice worker with a multi-dimensional view of patients' circumstances, allowing the advice worker to triangulate three sources of information (i.e. patient input, GP perspective and medical histories). It also acted as the catalyst for continuous engagement between the advice worker and GPs, and the collaborative production of supporting medical statements for health-related benefits.

Access to such information was a fundamental factor in creating a parity of professionalism between GPs and the advice worker, whose preparation of draft medical statements could only be achieved in this way. This approach reduces the workload of GPs, but still requires their expert medical knowledge, as they ultimately sign off any supporting evidence before final submission.

This process strengthened relationships between the two parties, through regular engagement and communication regarding the individual circumstances of people accessing the service. It also removed any potential for a hierarchical relationship to develop, as both professionals drew upon their respective expertise and knowledge to support people using the social security system.

In comparison, during the same 17-month period, the other 42 general practices in northeast Glasgow (without embedded advice workers but able to refer patients via an online system) made only 24 referrals to GEMAP's service.

Our findings suggest that a key feature underpinning the difference in referral figures (and GP engagement) is the development of familiarity and trust between a single financial advice worker and two practices, with each respecting the other's knowledge and expertise.

14.2.7 Building connections: Street-level evaluation and analysis

During the delivery phase of the project, a colleague from Building Connections (JS) regularly visited the general practices. Through conducting real-time evaluation and analysis of quantitative data (e.g. referrals, financial impact) and feeding this information back to practitioners, this approach aimed to identify opportunities to improve the project as it developed.

Through frequent visits and short, yet focused, conversations with all practitioners and practice staff, JS developed a robust understanding of the mechanisms underpinning the project and the experiences of practice staff. These understandings were used to support partners and identify opportunities to improve the referral processes and the delivery of the advisory services.

The availability and regular presence of this third party ensured that every individual involved in the project had the opportunity to articulate their experience and contribute to its development. He also acted as an additional resource 'on the ground', supporting practitioners to work through the complexities inherent in collaborative service delivery projects.

14.2.8 The importance of practitioner knowledge

Although there were clear differences between the two practices, in terms of their patient caseloads and service delivery structures, the knowledge of practice staff and advice worker was consistently positioned and used as a fundamental source of expertise.

Our experience makes clear that building embedded models of service delivery demands that the experiences and knowledge of practitioners are central in their design, delivery and ongoing development. Through understanding, valuing and acting upon the experiences of people practically involved in delivering and supporting the project, the Deep End Advice Worker Project efficiently and regularly implemented changes to its supporting mechanisms to test whether a better delivered and experienced service could be achieved.

14.2.9 Conclusion

The Deep End Advice Worker Project makes explicit the importance of the universal nature and trusted status of general practices in increasing the reach of advice services. Put simply, anyone can attend their local practice. People also tend to have longstanding and positive relationships with their GPs. These elements of trust and familiarity offer the opportunity to improve the accessibility and uptake of support services, particularly by those who may not otherwise use mainstream services.

The project sought to minimise barriers to accessing the service. For example, the advice worker delivered advice from a consultation room in each practice and mirrored the traditional GP call for attendance when people were waiting in the practice waiting room. In this way, the nature of the work carried out by the advice worker was kept discrete.

The project is now working from nine general practices in the surrounding area. Further work is needed to extend the approach to other geographic areas, with specific consideration of communities disproportionately affected by poverty, such as carers, lonely parents and ethnic minority communities.

It is fundamental that colleagues involved in the delivery of future projects of this nature appreciate the unique context, histories and demographics of their own workplaces and the communities they serve. The project is not prescriptive but, rather, highlights a set of principles or approaches which could be utilised in other locations.

REFERENCES

14 Introduction

1. Massie RK. *Catherine the Great: Portrait of a Woman.* Head of Zeus, London, UK, 2012, p. 340.
2. Hart JT assisted by Davey Smith G. Response rates in South Wales 1950–96: Changing requirements for mass participation in human research. In Non-random reflections on Health Services Research. Maynard A, Chalmers I (Eds). Nuffield Trust 1997, pp 31–57.
3. Watt GCM, Foy CJW, Hart JT. Comparison of blood pressure, sodium intake and other variables in offspring with and without a family history of high blood pressure. *Lancet* 1983;321(8336):1245–1248.
4. Watt GCM, Edwards C, Foy CJW, Hart JT, Hart M, Walton P. Dietary sodium restriction for mild hypertension in general practice. *British Medical Journal* 1983;286:432–436.
5. Watt GCM, Foy CJW, Hart JT, Bingham G, Edwards C, Hart M, Thomas E, Walton P. Dietary sodium and arterial blood pressure: Evidence against genetic susceptibility. *British Medical Journal* 1985;291:1525–1528.

14.1 Rules of engagement

1. Mercer SW, Watt, GCM, Maxwell M, and Heaney DH. The development and preliminary validation of the consultation and relational empathy (CARE) measure: An empathy-based consultation process measure. *Family Practice* 2004;21(6):699–705.
2. Mercer SW, O'Brien R, Fitzpatrick B, Higgins M, Guthrie B, Watt G, Wyke S. The development and optimisation of a primary care-based whole system complex intervention (CARE Plus) for patients with multimorbidity living in areas of high socioeconomic deprivation. *Chronic Illness* 2016;12(3):165–181.

14.2 Deep End Advice Worker Project

1. Sinclair J. Building Connections: Co-locating advice services in general practices and job centres. Glasgow Centre for Population Health. December 2017. Downloadable from info@gcph.co.uk.

15

Evaluation

How could they tell?

Dorothy Parker
(on being told of the death of President Calvin Coolidge)

Decisions in health care usually draw on experience, are sometimes based on evidence but are always underpinned by values. In many ways, health care systems are an expression of societal values, including the strengths of interest groups and their ability to command power and resource. Evidence can challenge the distribution of power and resource, but change is more likely when interests are aligned.

Many of the projects and activities described in this book stemmed from the collective imagination, enthusiasm and energy of the participants. There was little need to convince others, which was often as well, given the lack of resource for rigorous evaluation.

Evaluation can serve two main purposes. Internal evaluation establishes whether and how a project is working. For emergent activities learning by trial and error, which is the norm for customising initiatives to local circumstances, ongoing internal evaluation can speed up the process (See Section 14.2). External evaluation is chiefly concerned with whether a project works and provides value for money. How it works and identification of active ingredients are secondary considerations. All of this information is needed if others are to be persuaded to fund and repeat the initiative elsewhere.

In the case of link workers (Chapter 8), the Scottish Government committed to an expansion of the scheme, with 250 new posts, before its formal evaluation had been completed – but that is another story.

In this section, Sanjeev Sridharan reflects and looks ahead to the challenges of evaluating developments in primary care such as the "Deep End." Drawing on his extensive international experience of health care and health system evaluation, he first provides "thoughts from abroad" on what needs to be learned from the Deep End Project and then sets out a more general framework for evaluating developments in primary care.

If you truly want to understand something, try to change it.

Kurt Lewin

15.1 LEARNINGS FROM THE DEEP END

SANJEEV SRIDHARAN

As described in the introduction of this book: 'To counter the dominance of specialism in health care, generalist clinical care needs a competing narrative based on solutions to the health care challenges of multimorbidity, fragmented care, increased pressure on emergency services and static inequalities in health'.

Evaluation can be defined both as a means of assessing performance and as a means of identifying alternative means of delivery. For example, the Canadian Federal Evaluation Policy developed by the Treasury Board of Canada defines evaluation as 'the systematic collection and analysis of evidence on the outcomes of programmes to make judgments about their relevance, performance and alternative ways to deliver them or to achieve the same results'.

The question I ask is: What roles can evaluation play in locating the clinical generalist role in addressing multimorbidity and other health care challenges as highlighted above?

The question can be answered narrowly by focusing on evaluations of specific service developments related to general practice, but there is also a richer, more comprehensive view of the role of evaluations. In the broader 'ecology of care,' especially the care that relates to multimorbidity, what are the specific contributions of general practice?

Box 15.1 states the three building programmes that are important to realise the exceptional potential of general practice. Evaluation can help to clarify the role of general practice in each programme. Taking a system view to evaluation can also highlight the role of other components of the ecology of the health system (including narrow specialisms) in realising the full potential of general practice.

> **BOX 15.1: Three building programmes to realize the exceptional potential of general practice**
>
> A. Building strong patient narratives based on knowledge and confidence in living with their conditions and making good use of available services and resources
> B. Building the capacity of local health systems based on general practice hubs linked to local services and resources for health
> C. Building general practice as a whole system to ensure that "the best anywhere becomes the standard everywhere"

The Deep End Project (comprising the collective activities of general practitioners at the Deep End and referred to below as "Deep End") provides a case study on the role of general practice in delivering health care in very deprived areas. Evaluation of the Deep End would need to include both a project and·a system perspective. The project perspective focuses on the narrower details of what was learned from participating general practices. The system perspective focuses on the learnings that need to be spread more widely in Scotland and beyond.

15.1.1 A brief introduction to Deep End

Deep End is based on the deceptively simple idea that creating an ongoing dialogue space, in which there are opportunities to learn from the experiences and insights of the GPs, can help with the transformation of the health system.

It is perhaps useful to view Deep End as an innovation because as far as I am aware there is not an evidence base on how dialogue between practitioners working in 'Deep End' communities can transform local health systems. Deep End was developed as a dialogue space, an academic-service collaboration and a systematic attempt to capture what was said in dialogues to inform a common view, lobby for change and set up demonstration projects. This might be one of the first times that a dialogue space and the other activities described above have been implemented to help map and learn from the heterogeneous experiences of Deep End practitioners.

Many of the above statements need to be carefully challenged and interrogated, for example, the notion that dialogue between general practitioners can transform local health systems is in itself an assumption. Evaluations need to test such assumptions.

The Deep End Project has generated a rich set of learnings that have been discussed in a series of articles in the *British Journal of General Practice* (see Box 15.2).

Whether such learnings have transformed local practices involved in the Deep End or transformed the health system need focused evaluation.

Despite the excitement of such achievements, there is little reason why any of this will be more than episodic if there is not a focus on spreading, sustaining or mainstreaming the learnings.

BOX 15.2: Selective examples of learnings from the Deep End Project (1)

- Raise awareness of the importance of moving away from one-shot episodic interventions towards systemic sustainable solutions in Deep End communities;
- The need to move beyond a narrow view of evidence-based medicine and the need for an unconditional approach to addressing needs;
- Raise questions regarding the need for different performance metrics of performance based on the workload to address the needs of patients with complex needs;
- A better understanding of the dynamics of prevention and learnings about which "groups" to target from a long-term dynamic perspective;
- The need for intersectoral approaches and continuous, coordinated processes to address the needs of individuals with complex problems;
- Enhanced understanding of the connectedness of health and social problems in deprived communities;
- Clarify the role of GPs in social prescribing;
- Enhanced understanding of GP needs, e.g. extra time for consultation;
- Enhanced emphasis on the need for political action on alcohol;
- Raise focused questions regarding the limited effectiveness of brief interventions (and the need for collaborative sustainable solutions);
- A better understanding of the complexities of clients living in the Deep End communities;
- Clarify the role of GPs in joined up solutions;
- Enhanced focus on the need for solutions that understand the concentrated nature of poverty;
- Developing knowledge about (i) best use of serial encounters; (ii) the need for better connections across the front line; (iii) better support for the front line;
- Development of a community of GPs;
- Development of new interventions that respond to the needs of the disadvantaged communities;
- Developing knowledge of interventions in Deep End communities that might not work in the poorest communities—as an example, information delivered through pamphlets is unlikely to be effective.

15.1.2 Some examples of evaluation questions applied to the Deep End Project

Next, I briefly describe some of the evaluation questions that can help realize the potential of the learnings from the Deep End Project. Only a small set of questions are raised to highlight the value added of evaluative thinking.

a. **How is the Deep End likely to impact local practices and the health system in Scotland? Towards a theory of change**
   The theory of change that connects Deep End activities to improvements in local systems and the health system is still unclear. One important role for the evaluation will be to clarify how Deep End activities and ideas can impact health outcomes in disadvantaged communities, both within Deep End communities and more widely. The evaluation itself has a role in helping to bring about greater clarity on the nature of Deep End interventions over time.

   While Deep End has helped to develop and sustain a dialogue, it is important to recognise that dialogue is only the initial trigger of the process. A number of other ingredients are the key to the Deep End Project impacting local practices and health systems in Scotland. This impact might only emerge over time.

   A key starting point is to explore whether and how implementations of Deep End learnings can make a difference to the health of individuals living in Deep End communities?. Such a theory of change needs to pay great attention to the heterogeneous needs of individual patients. It would need to consider how recommendations can be spread beyond the participating Deep End practices. It would need to describe processes by which there is buy-in for Deep End recommendations from national-level policymakers with a genuine commitment to implement and sustain learnings from Deep End more widely. Given the focus on multimorbidity, a theory of change needs to pay great attention to the multiple mechanisms by which Deep End recommendations can address the challenges of multimorbidity.

b. **What can we learn from the evidence base to clarify the programme theory of Deep End?**
   One way in which knowledge translation can be strengthened is by leveraging the evidence base to further develop the theory of change of Deep End. The focus of the evidence review should be on clarifying the theory of change, and in particular the mechanisms by which dialogue spaces can lead to action. Such review should help develop a theory of change including the intermediate steps by which bringing general practices together can make a difference to health outcomes.

c. **What do we need to learn from the evaluation of Deep End? Where are the key gaps/uncertainties in our learning?**
   An evaluation needs to make explicit the uncertainties in the theory of change. Care needs to be taken that the evaluation is not used purely to

validate known solutions but also to generate a new set of questions that highlight areas of uncertainty in the theory. Possible learnings from an evaluation might include:

Policy learning: How exactly does Deep End fit into the inequities agenda in Scotland? What can be learned from the evaluation for future policy in Scotland?

Organizational learning: What changes need to be made in primary care services in the most deprived communities? What specific support services are needed in the most deprived practices to improve the effectiveness of GPs?

Barriers: Better understanding of what makes primary care different in Deep End communities as compared to other areas of Scotland; develop better knowledge of the heterogeneous lives of individuals living in Deep End communities; help identify suitable points of intervention given the complexity of patients' lives.

Process learning: How can knowledge developed from the Deep End dialogues be translated into well-defined interventions? What structures and processes are necessary to support such knowledge translation?

Impact learning: What are the impacts of Deep End? Is there evidence that patients' lives are improving as a result of implementing Deep End learnings?

d. **How do we know if Deep End has been a success? What are the impacts of Deep End?**

This step is the heart of the evaluation. An evaluation design is needed to assess if the Deep End Project has been successful. In all likelihood, some sort of a 'quasi-experiment' needs to be implemented to study the difference Deep End makes over time to:

- Deep End communities
- General practitioners
- Individuals living in Deep End communities
- Other communities in Scotland

The design needs to be informed by:

- Definitions of what success means at each of the above levels
- Theory of change
- Learning framework described above

In addition to assessing impacts, the evaluation design should help test critical assumptions underlying Deep End. An example of an assumption that might need to be tested includes whether there is buy-in for Deep End recommendations from stakeholders who are not GPs or who work outside Deep End communities. The design also needs to be able to study the unintended/unforeseen consequences of Deep End.

15.2 TOWARDS A FRAMEWORK OF LEARNING

SANJEEV SRIDHARAN

The previous section highlighted some of the ways in which thinking evaluatively about Deep End can be helpful. We now proceed to more general arguments of how evaluations can help with learning about the 'exceptional potential' of general practice. Once again it is useful to differentiate between learnings from specific interventions related to general practice (e.g. specific Deep End Projects) versus learnings that are possible from spreading and scaling up the project more widely (e.g. spreading learning from the Deep End Project across Scotland).

Figure 15.1 differentiates learnings from projects and learnings from spread initiatives.

15.2.1 Learnings from projects

i. **Process/Mechanisms**

Critical to the success of any project is the ability to activate mechanisms by which the project can impact on outcomes (1,2). An evaluation can be extremely helpful in learning about the mechanisms that are responsible for an intervention to achieve its effects.

Realist Evaluation (2) focuses on the mechanisms by which interventions achieve outcomes in specific contexts. Such an evaluation provides an opportunity to learn about such mechanisms and processes under a variety of contexts and support structures. For example, there needs to be a focus on the conditions under which a generalist approach is likely to be successful in 'Deep End' communities. The evaluation needs to highlight the support structures and the context necessary to realize the 'exceptional potential' of general practice.

ii. **Organizational Support Structures**

Interventions (even mainstreamed interventions) should be viewed as complex organizations thrust into other existing organizations (2). The likely success of interventions is increased by paying attention to the organizational structures necessary to achieve their effects. An evaluation can highlight the knowledge of organizational structures that are necessary for an intervention to achieve impacts.

Such organizational knowledge is especially important because interventions are often inserted into existing structures and cultures without attention to how these additional investments in personnel and other resources will connect/integrate/embed within the existing structures and cultures. Our experience in evaluating multiple interventions is that good programme

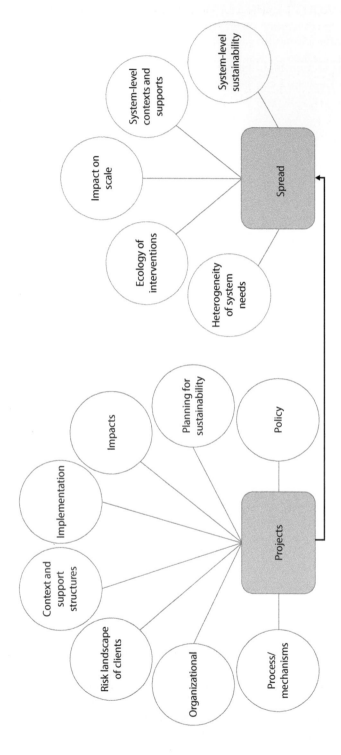

Figure 15.1 Some examples of learnings that are possible from evaluations.

planning requires knowledge of the organizational structures necessary for interventions to work.

One of the strengths of exploring the role of the clinical generalist is that generalists are already part of routine practice rather than part of an externally imposed intervention of a temporary kind. Although clinical generalists are part of routine practice, an evaluation can help generate knowledge of the supportive organizational structures necessary for clinical generalists to be successful.

iii. **Risk Landscape of Clients**

Projects such as the Deep End have the ambition of learning from the needs of the poorest individuals. Often knowledge of patients' needs is based not on deep knowledge of the lives of patients but on assumptions made about patients' lives without the knowledge of the constraints and barriers that individuals might face.

An evaluation provides an opportunity to learn about the lives and constraints of individuals that an intervention might hope to impact. We label this as the 'risk landscape' of patients because many of these risks might intersect with each other. An evaluation provides an opportunity to learn about such a risk landscape. One implicit claim in the 'exceptional potential' of general practice is that the general practitioner is in a better position to understand the risk landscape of patients. An evaluation needs to interrogate such a claim, by exploring if the patients believe that the general practitioner is curious, interested in and knowledgeable about their lives.

iv. **Implementation**

Evaluations can also provide opportunities to learn about how to implement interventions in specific contexts and settings. With the growth of the field of Implementation Science, there is an entire field that is focused on how best to implement interventions in specific settings. Evaluation provides an opportunity to learn how to navigate contextual barriers. There are multiple challenges with implementing interventions in different contexts, but this is especially true in contexts that are resource-poor and located in fragile settings. Spreading learnings from the Deep End Project widely across Scotland will require paying attention to implementation challenges. For example, in some contexts, there might not be the same 'buy-in' for the insights that have emerged from the Deep End Project.

v. **Impacts**

Clearly, one of the most important goals of evaluation is to help build knowledge of the impacts of an intervention. A variety of designs are typically implemented to learn about impacts.

Experimental and quasi-experimental designs are popular methods of learning about impacts in health care. The challenge is not just to learn about impacts from a specific design, but also how multiple evaluation designs can be combined to learn about the variety of questions associated with programme impacts? The questions might include: What specific components of an intervention are associated with programme impacts? What intervention mechanisms primarily drive the impact?

There can also be a set of impact questions related to equity. For example, do interventions disproportionately benefit the disadvantaged as compared to the well-off? An evaluation can help build knowledge of both overall impacts and differential impacts. A realist evaluation focuses on 'what works for whom under what conditions' (3). Additionally, in our experience, the impacts of existing routine practices are harder to study than the impacts of an externally imposed intervention that is being piloted.

vi. **Planning for Sustainability**

An intervention typically takes a long time to impact on outcomes such as inequities in health. Projects typically are funded for a short period, typically between one to five years. In order to maintain outcomes, however, projects have to plan for sustainability. An evaluation can help build knowledge of how programmes can best be integrated with existing organizational structures in order to mainstream and sustain the programme. In our experience, most programmes worry about sustainability when the funding is running out. There is a growing literature around sustainability that stresses that interventions need to plan upfront for sustainability. This literature stresses that planning for sustainability needs to precede an assessment of impacts – in fact, programme impacts are more likely to occur if interventions have planned for sustainability. One of the strengths of general practice is that sustainability is already built into its structure. Such a 'sustainability' dividend can contribute towards its exceptional potential.

vii. **Policy Learning**

A project such as Deep End is more likely to work if there are supportive policies. Projects and programmes are often of finite duration and implemented usually in specific settings. Policies, on the other hand, often have a provincial or national focus and are implemented for longer periods. An evaluation can help generate knowledge from projects of the types of policies that need to be in place to achieve population-level outcomes.

15.2.2 Learnings about spread

It's important to stress that learnings from projects often cannot simply be extrapolated, scaled up or spread to other contexts. For example, a programme might have worked very well in Glasgow, but decisions to generalise or scale up such programmes more broadly across Scotland need to be carefully made. To the extent that the focus is not just on a few individuals/practices who came into contact with the project, but on population-level outcomes, a focus is needed on what needs to be learned from a project to inform the spread of learnings/innovations from the project.

In our view, the learnings that are important to think about in spreading interventions include:

- **Heterogeneity of system needs**: Spreading learnings/innovations from projects depends critically on what might be the system-level needs across multiple contexts. The needs might differ across geographies, cultures, etc. A focus on spread needs to be guided by system-level needs.
- **An ecology of interventions**: An important idea of spread is that singular interventions often do not have sufficient leverage by themselves to achieve changes in complex outcomes. What may be needed are multiple interventions – perhaps an ecology of interventions. An evaluation framework focused on spread needs to pay attention to such knowledge of ecologies of interventions. The relevance of this idea is that the focus should be on the ecology of supports necessary for the general practice to thrive. It is possible that the 'exceptional potential' of general practice is unlikely to be realized without a supportive ecology.
- **Impacts on the scale**: An evaluation also needs to help learn whether if a project needs to be scaled up, it could still have impacts at scale. Often programmes that work in specific contexts may not achieve the same set of results at scale. Put differently, care needs to be taken to scale-up general practice interventions based on pilots in specific settings.
- **System-level contexts and support structures**: Another focus of evaluation can be on understanding the types of system-level supports needed to spread an intervention or to have impacts to scale. This is especially important because while initial projects may be well-endowed with external funding, it is important to build knowledge on the types of structures/supports needed at the national level to support scaling up/spread. While general practice is already routine, the question can hinge on the types of resources needed to provide needs-based care in Deep End communities – e.g. more time needed with complex patients.
- **System-level sustainability**: If some of the recommendations from Deep End do get scaled up, there needs to be knowledge of what it would take for them to be sustained and spread at the system level.

15.2.3 Conclusions

We have argued that evaluation approaches can help value the 'exceptional potential' of general practice. The value added of general practice can both be on its own and in conjunction with other practices/services. We have argued for an approach to evaluation that pays attention to what needs to be learned to establish value. Establishing the value of general practice would require engagement with patients themselves to establish how their diverse needs are being met and what needs to occur to better meet their needs. Such establishing of value can be aided by multiple evaluation approaches including summative (Is general practice working for you?), formative (How can general practice be improved?) and developmental (How can feedback from patients help develop new structures and systems to better serve their needs?) (4).

REFERENCES

15.1 Learnings from the Deep End

1. Watt G. General practitioners at the deep end: The experience and views of general practitioners working in the most severely deprived areas of Scotland. *Occas Pap R Coll Gen Pract* 2012;89(i–viii):1–40.

15.2 Towards a framework of learning

1. Pawson, R. *Evidence-Based Policy: A Realist Perspective*. London, UK: Sage, 2006.
2. Pawson, R. *The Science of Evaluation*. London, UK: Sage, 2013.
3. Pawson R. and Tilley N. *Realist Evaluation*. Thousand Oaks, CA: Sage, 1997.
4. Patton, M. *Developmental Evaluation: Applying Complexity Concepts to Enhance Innovation and Use*. New York: Guilford Press, 2010.

16

Education and training

Knowledge and wisdom, far from being one,
Have oft times no connexion : Knowledge dwells
In heads replete with thoughts of other men;
Wisdom in minds attentive to their own.
Knowledge is proud that he has learned so much.
Wisdom is humble that he knows no more.

William Cowper

16.1 CORRECTION OF SOCIAL IGNORANCE

For the time being, only a small minority of medical students have personal experience of the personal and working lives of most of their future patients, and intellectual opposition to social injustice, even when present, is only the beginning of understanding. If students are to retain patient-oriented rather than disease-oriented motivation, they must learn to identify in complex, concrete, detailed terms with people they know only as crude stereotypes and of whom they are usually afraid.

Ideal humane commitment to patients in general must be transformed into effective concern for real people; the present hierarchy of specialties that relegates primary care, geriatric and psychiatric care to the bottom of the heap shows that this transformation is hardly attempted by our present medical education, let alone achieved. Only after this phase of social re-education, it is safe to make the partial and the controlled detachment that is absolutely necessary to effective doctoring.

Primary care is a good level (though not the only one) at which to impart this unshared common social experience, to learn real rather than formal respect for patients, the many ways in which doctors must be subordinate to patients, and that the sick must become the subjects rather than the objects of care. This part of medicine has got to be rebuilt, and this may be best done by little doctors of slight authority, close and exposed to patients, with a minimum of technical and social armour (1).*

* Reprinted from Hart JT. Relation of primary care to undergraduate education. *Lancet* 1973;302:778–781.

16.2 A LIFELINE FOR A DROWNING MAN

JOHN FREY

I was finishing my family medicine residency training in Miami in 1973, after having been in medical school in Chicago in the late 1960s, immersed in the chaos and violence and energy of cities. The list of what I could do after residency was long, but my experience was short. I was offered a wonderful opportunity to work in a rural county in the mountains of North Carolina. I had never felt 'recruited' before but was simply grateful to have finished my education with an opportunity to practice my craft, to be a family doctor in a place that needed me. The cardiologist who came to see us in our residency made the case for his underserved rural community's need for general practitioners and flew three of us to his small town for a visit.

In addition to the soft beauty of the Appalachian mountains and the kindness and dedication of the cardiologist and his family, I remember the evening they arranged with community leaders and faculty members from the local college, who discussed their teaching, their research interests and their lives working with students from those mountains who went on to become contributors to life and their communities. I realized then that the rewards of teaching, if not necessarily equal to those of doctoring, were compelling. Both required the same patience, commitment to small but important changes, and a lot of patting oneself on the back when no one was looking. I knew then that I wanted to combine the roles, somehow. But that was not going to happen in that community.

I got my first teaching post in a new medical school, a new residency training program, in a part of the United States where I had never lived. I bought the 'theory of possibilities' that the director of the program had presented – that we could create something from scratch, designing an educational program that was unconventional, grounded in values of service and community, and a program for which we could make the rules and structures. It was seductive and, at first at least, true.

But the pressure for educational standardisation began squeezing creativity and innovation from the program in the guise of quality. Since it began in the late 1960s, family medicine has been defensive about approval from the traditional educational hierarchy. So, after designing community-responsive education programs in the early years, family medicine quickly adopted the look of traditional residency programs, with a standard curriculum emphasising hospital and procedural training, the technical before the behavioural, and a focus on individuals rather than context. My initial enthusiasm and energy for educational reform ran head-on into the reality of bureaucratic intransigence making me wonder if I might have chosen the wrong venue for my career or perhaps, even, the wrong field.

The Appalachian mountain community started to seem a lot more attractive to me. From the distance of time, I now realize that a periodic questioning of purpose is both normative and predictable. Without it, we risk what Jean Dubuffet called 'a long wearing away of oneself and eventual extinction' (1). But the first time that happened, I was both humbled and not a little discouraged. I also felt like I was drowning.

I had a colleague, in those days of paper journals, who was a regular reader of the *Lancet*. He put an article he tore from an issue from October 1973 in my box with the note 'thought you might find this interesting'. Not only was I interested, the article would change the trajectory of my career and life. The title was straightforward enough: 'Relation of Primary Care to Undergraduate Education' and it was written by Julian Tudor Hart, Glyncorrwg Health Centre, near Port Talbot, Glamorgan (2).

After reminding readers of where general practice started by referencing the Collings Report, the extraordinary narrative of the conditions of general practice at the start of the NHS, Julian wrote of the mission of new doctors from his now well-known perspective of a GP practicing in a coal mining village in South Wales, facing the legacy of teaching institutions that failed to train doctors for the task of building general practice.

He wrote that medical schools should be training 'a new generation of doctors for battle against what is unjust and intolerable in the service as it is, help them to become fearless, precise, and relevant in their criticism and mitigate such impudence by giving them a better technical training than the generation they displace'. I had found someone who articulated the reason I was willing to try to change medical education knowing the odds were slim – entering the 'battle' as Julian put it. How could a GP write with such eloquence about the mission of education from a village described as 'near' another larger town in Wales?

That article in my inbox led to an exploration of Julian's other published work and, after a long series of decisions about leaving where I started teaching, finding a new position in a school that I hoped would be more responsive and wanting to take a sabbatical of some sort – to explore what the NHS felt like on the ground. Soon my family and I were living in that Welsh village, practicing alongside Julian Tudor Hart and his staff, people who would become lifelong friends. I learned from them about combining hopefulness and tenacity in South Wales.

A decade and a half later, I had become the chair of a very large Department of Family Medicine in the United States and was trying to convey my vision of what I felt should be the values behind our work to my colleagues. I remembered what Julian had written in that article about the educational task of general practice and realized that what he recommended should also be our collective mission.

The first task was the correction of social ignorance to learn 'real rather than formal respect for patients, the many ways that doctors must be subordinate to patients, and that the sick must be the subjects rather than the objects of care.' Most students who arrive in medical schools still come with little experience with the daily lives and the struggles of their patients. Family doctors should be the guides for students to learn about the real lives of patients and communities.

A second task should be helping students and doctors in training learn to cope with uncertainty. Julian wrote of the limitations of the body of medical knowledge and of physicians, and the imprecision with which we practice despite endless research publications, evidence-based guidelines and narrower and more rarefied specialties.

The third task for general practice education, he wrote, should be training 'pioneers of new and better medical care' to practice in areas where they were needed the most – a trained and committed workforce that would begin to change the conditions in the Inverse Care Law. And these departments should be 'teaching a disciplined anger, not against people but against attitudes and situations that impede the effective delivery of medical science to sick people'. He finished by writing 'anger without discipline is mere cursing'.

When I first read that, I was 30 years old and my generation had just come through 15 years of the War in Vietnam, and civil rights. I had never thought of medical education as an incubator for careers dedicated to social justice! But Julian always has.

If there is a fundamental purpose for education in general practice, it still lies in the three tasks he outlined. Doctors and students are still ignorant of the lives of most of those for whom we provide care, the hunt for evidence and rigorous analyses of diagnosis and treatment collides with tradition, belief systems about medicine and patients who 'refuse' to improve despite the evidence that they should, and primary care, even as it struggles with becoming corporate and risks becoming more isolated from the lives of our patients still must be 'defining the intolerable, helping new generations to reject what we have bent to, and to express their rejection in great deeds and small words.' Those are the tasks that teachers in general practice and family medicine have to take as our responsibility and, through our work and with our example, pass that responsibility to subsequent generations.

16.3 THE SPECIAL NEEDS OF PRACTITIONERS WORKING IN DEPRIVED AREAS

AUSTIN O'CARROLL

When developing the North Dublin City GP Training Scheme (NDCGP), an interesting objection arose from a number of GPs and educators who felt that any graduate GP can work in an area of deprivation and that the development of a scheme with that specific focus would only serve to segregate the concept of social medicine to the minority of doctors willing to work in such conditions.

The belief that all doctors have adequate training to provide health care to all communities is rooted in the psycho-biophysical understanding of doctors as dispassionate scientists. It envisions the work of the medical practitioner as combating pathogens, managing disorders and reducing the risk of patients from dying at a young age from scientifically proven statistical risks. Once a practitioner has imbibed the clinical knowledge and learned the necessary diagnostic and therapeutic skills, they can work in any corner of the battlefield. In areas of deprivation, there may be a higher preponderance of clinical foes to engage with, but the medical weapons and martial arts remain the same. Hence, we can produce standardised combat-ready doctors with a standardised training package.

This argument totally misses out on the importance of social context. The nature of general practice changes fundamentally as one changes the social context. The joys and tribulations of working in an isolated rural practice are different from those of working in an inner-city practice. The burden of illness may or may not be similar, but the social context of the differing localities creates significant disparities over a large range of factors e.g. the nature of those illnesses/conditions; how those illnesses impact on the daily lives of patients; the support provided by family and communities; the resources available within those communities; the health-seeking behaviours of patients; the educational and life skills possessed by members of these differing communities; and the hope and belief that as citizens they have a reasonable expectation and/or right to have a healthy life.

When it comes to marginalised populations, these differences become magnified e.g. many homeless people suffer inordinate levels of disease, often related to drug misuse; have no support from family and are disconnected from their community; have poor access to community resources; often avoid seeking medical help till their symptoms are fulminating and overpowering; have poor education and life skills; and possess little hope of having a healthier life and no conception of having a right to a healthy life.

The second argument relates to the first, in that it does not recognise that the nature of general practice can vary widely between social contexts and as such General Practitioners require differing clinical, management and communication skills for each context. Equipping doctors to work optimally in difficult social contexts such as in areas of poverty or with marginalised populations is not creating a segregated system but rather enabling doctors to provide a higher quality of health care in these areas and so help to reduce health inequities. This prevents a segregation between high-quality health care in high-income areas versus run-down and low-morale general practices for their neighbours in areas of deprivation.

16.4 GP TRAINING IN THE DEEP END

DAVID BLANE

> In the varied topography of professional practice, there is a high, hard ground overlooking a swamp. On the high ground, manageable problems lend themselves to solution through the use of research-based theory and technique. In the swampy lowlands, problems are messy and confusing and incapable of technical solution. The irony of this situation is that the problems of the high ground tend to be relatively unimportant to individuals or society at large, however great their technical interest may be, while in the swamp lie the problems of greatest human concern.

> **Donald Schon (1)**

The NHS should be at its best where it is needed most, or inequalities in health will widen. There is a large body of research that demonstrates the social gradient in health needs, with a two to three-fold increase (in premature mortality, the presence of physical and mental multimorbidity, or self-reported health) between the most affluent decile of the population and the least affluent decile (2,3). Yet, the distribution of GP resource is more or less flat across the population. This Inverse Care Law (4) – the difference between what GPs can do and what they could do if resourced according to the health needs of their practice populations – is a fundamental barrier to improve the quality and the volume of GP training in the Deep End.

But there are at least three other challenges related to GP education and training in areas of deprivation: the distribution of training (with implications for recruitment); the demands of the work (with implications for practitioner wellbeing and patient safety); and the nature of the evidence base (with implications for decision making).

First, in keeping with the Inverse Care Law, there is an 'Inverse Training Law', whereby there are considerably more GP training practices in more affluent areas compared to more deprived areas (5).

This is partly explained by the higher proportion of smaller, often single-handed, practices in deprived areas, which makes it more difficult to accommodate training requirements (6). The potential consequence of this unequal distribution of training experience is that trainees may feel less confident about working in Deep End practices if they have not had any exposure to them during their training (7).

A second challenge is related to the particular demands – on trainees and trainers – of working in deprived areas, as articulated in Deep End Report 7, summarising the views and experience of GP trainers in Deep End Practices (8). These demands relate to the high prevalence of health and social complexity alongside a greater likelihood of 'unworried unwell' patients with low health literacy and other barriers to engagement with health services (9).

Research comparing GP stress levels in practices serving deprived compared to affluent areas demonstrated increasing stress as consultation length increased in deprived areas but not in affluent areas – if you are having a challenging consultation and starting to run late in a deprived area, there is a high chance that the waiting room is filling up with equally complex patients (10).

The third challenge relates to the content of training. Given the particular nature of clinical work in deprived areas, characterised by high volumes of alcohol and drugs misuse, multimorbidity, psychological distress, polypharmacy, child protection issues and social problems, there are particular learning needs of GP trainees working in Deep End practices. These issues were highlighted in Deep End Report 24 (11) and a subsequent research paper (12) that summarised a roundtable discussion on the learning needs of Deep End GPs. There were three areas identified as having learning resource gaps:

- How to address low patient engagement in health care and increase health literacy.
- How to promote and maintain therapeutic optimism when working in areas of high deprivation.
- How to use Evidence-Based Medicine (EBM) effectively when working with patients with high levels of multimorbidity and social complexity.

The third area merits particular consideration. How generalisable is the 'evidence' derived from trials that routinely exclude Deep End patients (either due to comorbidities or difficulties in recruiting to trials)? How applicable to Deep End general practice are the guidelines that this evidence informs?

This section has highlighted some of the fundamental challenges of GP training in the Deep End. The question of whether and how the content of training covers the sorts of knowledge, skills and attitudes needed to address multimorbidity and social complexity in Deep End general practice is harder to answer. The next sections describe initiatives to improve GP recruitment and retention in areas of material deprivation, with a particular focus on doctors' learning needs.

16.5 THE NORTH DUBLIN CITY GP TRAINING SCHEME (NDCGP)

AUSTIN O'CARROLL

In the early 2000s, North Dublin provided a clear demonstration of Tudor Hart's Inverse Care Law. Despite having large tracts of deprivation with their attendant poor health indices, the GP to patient ratio was 1:2500, comparing poorly with the national ratio of 1:1600 (1). North Dublin also contained many members of marginalised groups (ethnic minorities, travellers, homeless, etc.) who had even worse access to primary and secondary health care (2–7). The final insult was that North Dublin had no GP training scheme compared to three in the more affluent south side of the city.

The North Dublin City GP Training Programme (NDCGP) was founded to address this imbalance. It is the first GP training scheme internationally that specifically trains GPs to work in areas of deprivation and with marginalised groups. Funding for the scheme was obtained by steadfastly (over several years) presenting the evidence-based argument for a GP training programme with a focus on social medicine and awaiting the opportunity when further funding was released to expand GP training. This coalescence of persistence and opportunity occurred in 2009.

Vision and Mission statements are the engines for everything we do.

16.5.1 Vision

Every person and community has access to a professional, quality and holistic general practitioner service that will allow them to maximise their health, irrespective of background and economic status.

16.5.2 Mission

To form professional and high-quality general practitioners whose passion is to maximise patient and community health in a holistic manner and whose own health is maximised through the ability to self-care.

The curriculum is designed to equip trainees with the highest standards in clinical and communication skills as our mission demands high-quality GP graduates. The social medicine modules furnish trainees with the knowledge and attitudinal skills to overcome stigma, address health inequalities, understand community approaches to health and advocate for both individual patients and communities affected by deprivation and marginalisation.

Patients in such communities have a high prevalence of psychological problems, so our graduates require context-specific knowledge and skills in order to manage complexity and uncertainty together (8). Trainees need to learn the art of collaborative work with other community agencies that address the determinants of health (9,10). Advocacy is an essential skill to help maximise the health of disenfranchised patients and communities (9). Current educational programmes that do not respond to these needs may be exacerbating the poor distribution of GPs in areas of deprivation (8,11,12).

As we believe that our trainees will change the world, we teach them change management, research and presentation skills. As we want to ensure graduates have the necessary resilience to work in the chaotic environment that often exists in communities of deprivation and marginalization, we have developed a self-care programme. This includes developing a personal self-care plan, participating in a mindfulness-based stress reduction programme and addressing the psychodynamics of the consultation through such approaches as Balint Groups or sessions on managing uncertainty.

Our hospital training and GP posts are located in areas of deprivation with hospital and GP teachers who understand and support our ethos. Participating practices must demonstrate that they operate with a low threshold and do not exclude patients on the basis of background, race, and so on.

In our fourth year, we have developed a particular social medicine placement whereby trainees spend one day a week working firstly, in homeless primary care services, followed by drug treatment settings and finally, prisons and/or migrant services. These posts are critical in educating our graduates in how to work with marginalised groups. The posts seek firstly to address any underlying stigmatic attitudes trainees might have and help them develop skills to work with these populations. The conceptual basis for the posts derives from Alport's Contact hypothesis which posits that interpersonal contact between majority and minority groups is the best method of reducing prejudice. This contact must be interactional (13,14).

Traditional medical teaching, whereby a member of a minority group is brought into a group of medical students to describe their life experiences, does not satisfy the four key criteria for contact, that is, institutional support, acquaintance, equal status and cooperation (15).

An interesting outcome of the scheme's emphasis on Vision and Mission (V&M) is that the trainees felt they needed to make these more tangible and so themselves formed a V&M Committee to focus on practical projects. In 2014/2015, they created the first ever Irish Street Medicine conference, which is now an annual event attended by all health professionals working with homeless people. In 2015/2016, they developed a GP trainee-run-out-of-hours clinic in a homeless hostel. In 2016/2017, they launched an advocacy campaign highlighting the effects of the direct provision system on refugee health. This year, they are planning to implement quality improvement projects for homeless and migrant services.

Finally, the scheme has developed a postgraduate Continuing Medical Education and Mentoring Service to support graduates of the Programme as they establish themselves in practices in areas of deprivation or in services for those marginalised.

16.5.3 Is the scheme achieving its objectives?

Firstly, would anyone apply? Since its first year, the NDCGP has had the highest number of applications of any GP training scheme in the Republic of Ireland. This single fact is enough to destroy any notion that young doctors are cynical and focussed on comfort and money. They actually do want to make a difference. The scheme has become a beacon for young doctors interested in social medicine and receives many requests from pre- and postgraduate students to sit in with GP trainers and trainees.

Secondly, are graduates working in areas of deprivation and with marginalised groups? In a follow-up survey in 2018 of 37 doctors who had experienced the scheme, 35 were working full time or part time in practices serving deprived populations or marginalised groups.

Thirdly, has the introduction of the scheme caused systemic change? It has had both national and international repercussions. The Irish College of General Practitioners requisitioned the NDCGP to provide a new module on Social Medicine for its national GP training curriculum. They also adopted a policy document recognising that each GP training scheme needs to have the flexibility to develop educational responses to local needs.

Following these developments, several rural schemes are developing teaching sessions to address related health issues in the context of rural 'pocket' deprivation. Internationally, Manchester is developing a training scheme similar to the NDCGP (Section 6.4). The Deep End Project in Glasgow (Sections 7.2 and 16.7) has developed a GP Pioneer Scheme to improve recruitment and retention of GPs in deprived areas which was inspired by the NDCGP. Northern Ireland is exploring the option of introducing a pioneer scheme.

The NDCGP has also had several unexpected consequences, integrating with several other projects in Dublin.

Safetynet is a charity that along with its affiliated members provides health services to hard-to-reach groups including homeless people, migrants and asylum seekers nationally. Safetynet offers a number of positions to GP registrars for the social medicine module and has been able to significantly improve its service provision due to the presence of these GP trainees.

Curam Healthnet is a social enterprise focussed on developing GP practices in areas of deprivation. It was developed in response to the launch of the NDCGP to exploit the opportunity created to develop practices in such underserved areas as the NDCGP solved the recruitment dilemma for such an initiative.

The Partnership for Health Equity was formed by the NDCGP with the Health Services Executive and the University of Limerick and has been joined by the Irish

College of General Practitioners. Its focus is to create a platform where educators, practitioners, researchers and policymakers can work in unison to address health inequity. Trainees have contributed to research and policy projects conducted by the Partnership.

Lastly, the most interesting and unexpected outcome was the appointment of an Inclusion Health Consultant in St James Hospital, who along with her nurse helps make the hospital a more effective and hospitable institution for marginalised patients. The other main hospital in Dublin (Mater Misericordiae) has appointed a nurse to manage similar patients.

The NDCGP has taken the Social Determinants of Health Model from a peripheral lecture to the core of its educational activities. Sending young doctors with a pure biomedical philosophy to work with populations affected by deprivation or marginalization is setting them up for disappointment and ultimately cynicism. We believe that by nurturing an appreciation of and fascination with the complex interaction between patient illness, psychology and social context, we are providing them with a philosophy that will produce more self-fulfilled and effective general practitioners.

16.6 THE SOUTH WALES GP ACADEMIC FELLOWSHIP SCHEME

MEGAN BLYTH, HARRY AHMED AND KEVIN THOMPSON

General practice in Wales faces challenges similar to the rest of the United Kingdom. Workload has increased (1) despite some initially promising innovations in working practice (2,3). As patients are living longer with more comorbidities than before (4). general practice is having to manage a greater number of complex patients. Recruitment and retention of GPs is difficult, especially in rural and socially deprived communities. In 2015, five Welsh general practices closed, 18 were taken over by local health boards, and 58 were deemed to be 'at risk' of closure or take-over (5). These issues further exacerbate health inequalities, as relatively under-staffed and under-resourced general practices become less able to meet the needs of patients in socially deprived communities (6).

In 2001, Cardiff University and the Welsh Government set up the Academic Fellows scheme to help address some of the challenges faced by general practice in deprived former coal-mining communities in South-East Wales. The scheme employs enthusiastic, recently qualified GPs as Academic Fellows (AFs) for a two-year fixed-term period. AFs spend two days working as GPs attached to a practice in a socially deprived community and three days involved with teaching and research activities at Cardiff University. The scheme has two main aims. Firstly, to provide much-needed support to practices in these socially deprived communities, allowing GPs to develop and refine services to improve patient care. Secondly, to aid recruitment and retention of GPs by exposing new GPs to clinical work in deprived communities whilst supporting their professional development by providing opportunities and financial support for teaching, research and postgraduate study.

16.6.1 How does the scheme benefit the academic fellows?

The AFs work in the Division of Population Medicine at Cardiff University School of Medicine and receive support from academics with expertise in primary care, epidemiology, clinical trials, biostatistics, social science and health psychology. AFs are encouraged to pursue research and over 90% have published papers in peer-reviewed journals. To date, all AFs gained a postgraduate qualification on completion of the scheme. These included Master-level qualifications in Medical Education, Public Health and Business Administration, and diploma level qualifications in Epidemiology and Medical Statistics. AFs have made significant contributions to undergraduate medical student teaching. They have developed novel teaching methods and have won Cardiff University teaching prizes. Over 80% of previous AFs have continued to partake some academic work following completion of the scheme. This ranges from part-time sessional teaching commitments to full-time research roles funded through external Fellowships.

16.6.2 How does the scheme benefit the hosting general practice?

The AFs cover host GPs' clinical work for two days each week to allow them to undertake clinically important service improvements. The scheme has supported GPs to successfully complete innovative improvement projects which otherwise would not have been possible. We provide brief examples of three such projects below. All were initiated and completed by the host practice to address an important clinical need within their practice population.

In 2016, death rates related to drug misuse were higher in Cwm Taf Health Board in the South Wales Valleys than the Welsh average (7). Several practices used AF time to develop and pilot substance-misuse clinics. The most recent example resulted in a benzodiazepine reduction programme that ultimately led to a 60% reduction in benzodiazepine prescribing.

Wales has an estimated 70,000 people with undiagnosed type 2 diabetes (8). One practice used AF time to develop and pilot a targeted screening programme for individuals at high risk of diabetes, e.g. those with obesity or of South Asian descent. The practice screened and followed up all relevant patients over the age of 40 and diagnosed 28 patients with type 2 diabetes, who were then appropriately counselled and managed.

One contributor to the GP recruitment and retention problem in rural and socially deprived communities in Wales may be the relative lack of exposure of undergraduate medical students to work in these areas. Several practices have used AF time to develop processes and procedures that allow the practice to commit to regular medical student teaching. This can make the practice more attractive to GPs wishing to include some teaching in their clinical work and may influence the students' future choices in terms of work location.

16.6.3 Wider benefits of the scheme and future direction

To date, the scheme has supported 59 practices to develop services that address the needs of their patients and hopes to support many more practices through recent expansion resulting in AF schemes in South-West Wales and North Wales.

The scheme has employed 34 AFs, 62% of whom continue to work as GPs in socially deprived areas of Wales. This is a significant achievement as these areas struggle to recruit and retain GPs. The contribution of the scheme to recruitment and retention in these areas was recently summed up by a previous AF, who said, 'The practice in which I am now a partner is one of the practices I was on placement in during the scheme. I don't think this would have happened otherwise ... by working on placement with the scheme I realised how I would fit into the practice'.

16.7 THE DEEP END GP PIONEER SCHEME

DAVID BLANE

> Our system of medical education is still designed to produce community clinicians only as a by-product, an afterthought following a core curriculum designed by and for specialists. Its central aim remains the production of specialist excellence, unsullied by prior contact with the society it serves. It is training the wrong people, at the wrong time, in the wrong skills, and in the wrong place. The core curriculum for all doctors should be primary care: this should be taught where it is actually carried out, within communities; and the primary generalists produced in this way require not a year or two of rehabilitation in specialized vocational training, but a lifetime of in-service postgraduate study.

> **Tudor Hart, 1998 (1)**

In October 2016, the Deep End GP Pioneer scheme (Section 7.2) was launched with funding from the Scottish Government's GP Recruitment and Retention Fund. The challenges related to GP recruitment and retention in underserved areas have been described elsewhere (2), but a particular issue in Scotland is the higher proportion of older GPs (closer to retirement) in more deprived areas, suggesting that these workforce challenges are going to increase (3).

The Pioneer scheme aimed to develop and establish a change model for general practices serving very deprived areas (4), involving the recruitment of younger GPs (or fellows), the retention of experienced GPs, and their joint engagement in strengthening the role of general practice as the natural hub of local health systems.

Six early career GP fellows were recruited through a competitive interview process to work in six Deep End practices, providing additional clinical capacity and releasing time for experienced GPs to work on service development. The fellows also have protected time for professional and service development, with the aim that learning is shared between practices working as a non-geographical cluster.

The Fellow's protected time on Wednesdays alternates between attendance at day release sessions at the University Department of General Practice, and service development projects agreed with the GP lead at their respective practices.

The timetable for the day release sessions is organised by the Academic Co-ordinator and includes clinical learning (e.g. areas such as mental health, addictions) as well as broader learning in areas such as GP service development, preventing burnout and academic writing.

The content of the day-release sessions was based in part on the learning needs of Deep End GPs identified in Deep End Report 24 (5,6) and on a learning needs assessment of the GP fellows, and making use of existing contacts and networks.

The aim was to make the learning as grounded and practical as possible – ideally delivered by experienced Deep End GPs (some with a special interest, e.g. in child protection or addictions) or by other health and social care professionals who represent important interfaces with Deep End general practice (Table 16.1).

A key output of the day-release programme is documentation arising from the sessions, with the Deep End fellows as joint authors, comprising significant

Table 16.1 Pioneer scheme day-release curriculum

Session topic (Background of session lead)
Background to the Deep End Project (GP)
Multimorbidity (GP)
Inverse Care Law (GP)
Practitioner health / preventing burnout (GP)
Working in deprived areas (Group discussion)
Learning from Govan SHIP Project (GP)
Violence reduction (Police)
Domestic violence (NHS Health Scotland)
Adults with Incapacity (Group discussion)
Learning from Financial Inclusion Project (Third Sector, Building Connections)
Learning from the Links Worker Project (GP)
Managing difficult consultations (Clinical psychologist)
Leadership (Group discussion)
Multiple exclusion and complex consultations (GPwSI)[a]
Palliative care in the Deep End (GPwSI)[a]
End-of-life prescribing (Group discussion)
Asylum Health Bridging Team (Community Psychiatric Nurse from the AHBT)
Chronic pain and narrative (GP)
Trauma and shame (GP)
Living in poverty (Third Sector, Poverty Alliance)
Personality disorder and using mentalising in tricky GP consultations (Consultant psychiatrist and psychotherapist)

(Continued)

Table 16.1 (*Continued*) Pioneer scheme day-release curriculum

Session topic (Background of session lead)
Working with interpreters (Third Sector, Freedom from Torture)
Vulnerable families / child protection (GPwSI)[a]
Quality Improvement (Clinical Improvement, NHS)
Adult social work in the Deep End (Social Worker)
Addictions and Older Drug Users' health (Addictions)
Hepatitis (Third Sector, Hepatitis Scotland)
Social model of disability (Sociologist)
LGBT+ health inequalities (Paediatrician and Stonewall Ambassador)
Adolescent Health in the Deep End (Group discussion)
Homelessness/Destitution network (GPwSI)[a]
Female Genital Mutilation (GPwSI)[a]
Prisoner health (GPwSI)[a]
Visits to Keppoch Medical Practice (DE Fellows)

[a] GPwSI is a GP with a special interest.

learning in key areas, plus relevant reference materials and other resources. Fellows have dedicated time (approximately one session in alternate weeks) allocated to this task. The academic co-ordinator oversees and edits this output, which is shared online and through feedback sessions that the fellows have at their practices.

Other development opportunities have included:

- Joint teaching sessions with medical students (Student Selected Course in Social Determinants of Health)
- Presenting at the inaugural Deep End GP medical student conference
- Supporting school pupils applying to Medicine from SIMD20 schools via the REACH programme
- Teaching students from the Glasgow Access Programme (GAP)
- Representing the Deep End at conferences and meetings (e.g. RCGP Annual Conference, Regional Trainers Conference, Deep End meetings)

The Pioneer scheme has proven attractive to early-career GPs as it is a fellowship programme, which combines a supportive clinical environment with protected time for shared learning and leadership activities (7). While it is not a replacement for a 'lifetime of in-service postgraduate study,' the scheme has clearly demonstrated the impact that a small amount of protected time – something which has historically been unfunded and undervalued in UK general practice – can have.

Perhaps, the most successful aspect of the scheme has been its impact on GP retention. The older host GPs involved report a reduction in stress and renewed enthusiasm for their work, the result of a combination of additional clinical capacity provided by the fellows and their own protected time. We believe this model could be applied to other areas to support GP recruitment and retention.

16.7.1 A journey to the Deep End

Lisa Robins

I went to medical school as most 18-year olds do, full of ideas and an ambition to make the world a better place. Reality struck during a year at Leeds University doing a BSc in International Health, where I first learned about the wider determinants of health. During my foundation training in Glasgow, I realised that I wanted to work in general practice as I felt that I was seeing the same patients coming in and out of the wards, dealing only with their acute problems. We were then discharging them back to the care of their GPs, to the same complex environments, and with the same challenges.

I felt sure that there was a better way to tackle this. I swayed between public health and general practice training, deciding on the latter after realising that as a GP I could do both. My GP training was in a Deep End practice in Glasgow, in an area of pocket deprivation. After completing my training, I did GP locums for a year in both affluent and deprived areas and found that the work in Deep End practices was far more interesting and rewarding despite its many challenges. I was offered a job as a Deep End Pioneer Scheme Fellow in October 2016.

In my current role as a salaried GP in Possil (six sessions), I am getting to know my patients and the community in which they live. This is the longest time I have spent in one job as a doctor (a pro and con of our training system) and I am really enjoying the continuity. My skills in working with a very deprived, complex and multimorbid population are being developed and I am learning from experienced and enthusiastic GPs within a well-organised team (Section 7.2).

Our day release teaching sessions on alternate weeks have been invaluable and have covered a vast range of topics but have been targeted and highly relevant to working with deprived populations. Some of the topics covered so far include, for example, complex trauma, violence reduction, chronic pain, living in poverty, addiction and destitution. My own project/development time (two sessions on alternate weeks) has allowed me to work on audits (on migrant health and currently mental health referrals), writing (for reports, reflective diary, presentations and teaching) and sometimes just catching up on admin from clinical sessions, which reduces my stress levels on the days when I have surgeries.

I am part of the wider group of fellows, lead GPs and academic coordinators, between whom we share knowledge and provide support. I think this is one of the most important aspects of the scheme, particularly for the experienced GPs as they do not have the direct benefit of the day release group sessions.

Other than the perhaps predictable learning outcomes associated with the project, there have been a number of unexpected outcomes. Some of the preconceptions and prejudices that I often did not know I had have been challenged, particularly at the beginning. The process of the Pioneer Scheme itself has allowed me to learn more about funding, structures and processes within the NHS and some of the politics of health.

As well as being students again through the day release programme, I am learning new skills and gaining experience in teaching. This teaching has been both formal in presentations to medical and pre-medical students (on the Deep End, the pioneer scheme, alcohol and multimorbidity) and informal to school pupils (via the REACH programme) and to members of the practice team feeding back learning on day release topics at our weekly clinical meetings.

Getting to know my patients and learning about their potential needs have allowed me to be more of an advocate for them both on a day-to-day level and on a bigger scale when attending meetings at various levels (up to Scottish Government), which in itself is another new experience. My leadership skills have been developed a lot more quickly than if I had continued as a locum, or even as a salaried GP out with the scheme.

I feel that out of this pilot scheme and by becoming involved with the Deep End, I have become part of a movement that really puts patients at the heart of their practice and whose values, motivation and commitment are contagious. Already I feel like a more well-rounded doctor through it, and I am keen to continue working in the Deep End after the scheme, or at least my part in it, has ended. Crucially as an individual, I have learned more about the way in which I would like to work, and which I think is sustainable, in the future.

REFERENCES

16.1 Correction of social ignorance

1. Hart JT. Relation of primary care to undergraduate education. *Lancet* 1973;302:778–780.

16.2 A lifeline for a drowning man

1. Russell J. Jean Dubuffet, painter and sculptor, is dead. *New York Times*, May 15, 1985. /https://www.nytimes.com/1985/05/15/arts/jean-dubuffet-painter-and-sculptor-is-dead.html
2. Hart JT. Relation of primary care to undergraduate education. *Lancet* 1973:302:778–780.

16.4 GP training in the Deep End

1. Schön DA. *Educating the Reflective Practitioner: Toward a New Design for Teaching and Learning in the Professions.* San Francisco, CA: Jossey-Bass, 1987.
2. McLean G, Guthrie B, Mercer SW, Watt GCM. General practice funding underpins the persistence of the Inverse Care Law: Cross-sectional study in Scotland. *British Journal of General Practice* 2015; 65:e799–e805. doi:10.3399/bjgp15×687829.

3. Muldoon L, Rayner J, Dahrouge S. Patient poverty and workload in primary care: Study of prescription drug benefit recipients in community health centres. *Canadian Family Physician* 2013;59:384–390.
4. Hart JT. Inverse Care Law. *Lancet* 1971;297:405–412.
5. Russell M, Lough M. Deprived areas: Deprived of training? *British Journal of General Practice* 2010;60:846–848.
6. Blane DN, Hesselgreaves H, McLean G, Lough M, Watt GCM. Attitudes towards health inequalities amongst GP trainers in Glasgow, and their ideas for changes in training. *Education for Primary Care* 2013;24:97–104.
7. Crampton PE, McLachlan JC, Illing JC. A systematic literature review of undergraduate clinical placements in underserved areas. *Medical Education* 2013;47:969–978.
8. DEEP END REPORT 7 General practitioner training in very deprived areas, June 2010. Available from www.gla.ac.uk/deepend.
9. Dixon-Woods M, Kirk D, Agarwal S. Vulnerable groups and access to health care: A critical interpretive synthesis. London, UK: National Co-ordinating Centre for NHS Service Delivery and Organisation, 2005.
10. Mercer SW, Watt GCM. The Inverse Care Law: Clinical primary care encounters in deprived and affluent areas of Scotland. *Annals of Family Medicine* 2007;5:503–510.
11. DEEP END REPORT 24 What are the CPD needs of GPs working in Deep End practices? June 2014. Available from www.gla.ac.uk/deepend.
12. MacVicar, R., Williamson, A., Cunningham, D., Watt, G. What are the CPD needs of GPs working in areas of high deprivation? Report of a focus group meeting of 'GPs at the Deep End'. *Education for Primary Care* 2015;26:139–145. doi:10.1080/14739879.2015.11494332.

16.5 The North Dublin City GP Training Scheme (NDCGP)

1. Northern Area Health Board. *A Review of General Practice Manpower, Training, Recruitment and Retention*. Dublin, Ireland: Northern Area Health Board, 2000.
2. O'Carroll A, O'Reilly F. Health of the homeless in Dublin: Has anything changed in the context of Ireland's economic boom? *European Journal of Public Health* 2008;18:448–453. doi:10.1093/eurpub/ckn038.
3. O'Reilly F, Barror S, Hannigan A, Scriver S, Ruane L, McFarlane A, O'Carroll A. Homelessness: An unhealthy state. Health status, risk behaviours and service utilisation among homeless people in two Irish cities. Dublin: The Partnership for Health Equality, 2015.
4. All Ireland Traveller Health Study Team; School of Public Health, Physiotherapy and Population Science, University College Dublin. All-Ireland Traveller Health Study summary of findings. Dublin: Department of Health and Children, 2010.
5. Baggett TP, O'Connell JJ, Singer DE, Rigotti NA. The unmet health care needs of homeless adults: A national study. *American Journal of Public Health* 2010;100:1326–1333. doi:10.2105/AJPH.2009.180109.

6. Lebrun-Harris LA, Baggett TP, Jenkins DM, Sripipatana A, Sharma R, Hayashi AS, Daly CA, Ngo-Metzger Q. Health status and health care experiences among homeless patients in federally supported health centers: Findings from the 2009 patient survey. *Health Services Research* 2013;48:992–1017. doi:10.1111/1475-6773.12009.

7. Ware J, Mawby R. Patient access to general practice: Ideas and challenges from the front line. *Royal College of General Practitioners* 2015.

8. Riva M, Curtis SE. Long-term local area employment rates as predictors of individual mortality and morbidity: A prospective study in England, spanning more than two decades. *Journal of Epidemiology and Community Health* 2012;66:919–926.

9. Babbel, BE. Tackling health inequalities in primary care: An exploration of GPs' experience at the frontline. 2016 PhD thesis. Available from http://theses.gla.ac.uk/7692/.

10. Craven MA, Allen CJ, Kates N. Community resources for psychiatric and psychosocial problems: Family physicians' referral patterns in urban Ontario. *Canadian Family Physician* 1995;41:1325–1335.

11. Lambert T, Goldacre M. Trends in doctors' early career choices for general practice in the UK: Longitudinal questionnaire surveys. *British Journal of General Practice* 2011;61:e397–e403.

12. Thistlethwaite JE, Kidd MR, Hudson JN. General practice: A leading provider of medical student education in the 21st century? *Medical Journal of Australia* 2007;187:124–128.

13. Buchanan D, Rohr L, Kehoe L, Glick S, Jain S. Changing attitudes toward homeless people: A curriculum evaluation. *Journal of General Internal Medicine* 2004;19:566–568.

14. Knecht T, Martinez LM. Humanizing the homeless: Does contact erode stereotypes? *Social Science Research* 2009;38:521–534.

15. Brown R. *Prejudice: Its Social Psychology*. Oxford, UK: Blackwell, 2006.

16.6 The South Wales GP Academic Fellow Scheme

1. Hobbs FDR, Bankhead C, Mukhtar T et al. Clinical workload in UK primary care: A retrospective analysis of 100 million consultations in England, 2007-14. *Lancet* 2016;387:223–230. doi:10.1016/s0140-6736(16)00620-6.

2. Campbell JL, Fletcher E, Britten N et al. Telephone triage for management of same-day consultation requests in general practice (the ESTEEM trial): A cluster-randomised controlled trial and cost-consequence analysis. *Lancet* 2014;384:1859–1868. doi:10.1016/s0140-6736(14)61058-8.

3. Newbould J, Abel G, Ball S et al. Evaluation of telephone first approach to demand management in English general practice: Observational study. *British Medical Journal* 2017;358:j4197. doi:10.1136/bmj.j4197.

4. Barnett K, Mercer SW, Norbury M et al. Epidemiology of multimorbidity and implications for health care, research, and medical education: A cross-sectional study. *Lancet* 2012;380:37–43. doi:10.1016/s0140-6736(12)60240-2.
5. GP Wales heat map, British Medical Association, https://www.bma.org.uk/collective-voice/committees/general-practitioners-committee/gpc-wales (Accessed 30/01/18 12:17).
6. Mercer SW, Guthrie B, Furler J, Watt GCM, Hart JT. Multimorbidity and the Inverse Care Law in primary care. *British Medical Journal* 2012;344:e4152.
7. Substance Misuse, Drug deaths in Wales 2016, Public Health Wales. Available from http://www.wales.nhs.uk/sitesplus/documents/888/Drug %20related%20deaths%202016%20%20analysis%20of%20data%20from%20Office%20for%20National%20Sta....pdf (Accessed 30/01/18 10.43).
8. Diabetes UK. Available from https://www.diabetes.org.uk/in_your_area/wales/diabetes-in-wales (Accessed 30/1/18 at 10.29).

16.7 The Deep End GP Pioneer Scheme

1. Hart JT. George Swift lecture. The world turned upside down: proposals for community-based undergraduate medical education. *Journal of the Royal College of General Practitioners* 1985;35(271):63–68.
2. Crampton PE, McLachlan JC, Illing JC. A systematic literature review of undergraduate clinical placements in underserved areas. *Medical Education* 2013;47:969–978.
3. Blane DN, McLean G, and Watt G. Distribution of GPs in Scotland by age, gender and deprivation. *Scottish Medical Journal* 2015;60:214–219.
4. Blane DN, Sambale P, Williamson AE, Watt GCM. A change model for general practice in deprived areas, *Annals of Family Medicine* 2017;15:277.
5. DEEP END REPORT 24 What are the CPD needs of GPs working in deep end practices? June 2014. Available from www.gla.ac.uk/deepend.
6. MacVicar R, Williamson A, Cunningham D, Watt G. What are the CPD needs of GPs working in areas of high deprivation? Report of a focus group meeting of 'GPs at the Deep End'. *Education for Primary Care* 2015;26:139–145.
7. DEEP END REPORT 28 GP recruitment and retention in deprived areas. April 2016. Available from www.gla.ac.uk/deepend.

17

Preparations ahead of time

The outcome of any venture depends on preparations made ahead of time.

J. P. Morgan

An underlying theme mentioned by several contributors to this book is that professional teams are better able to look after others if they also look after their own well-being. This section reflects on how this challenge was addressed in the Department of General Practice at the University of Glasgow.

Although he died prematurely, the late Stuart Wood had already completed a quarter of a century as a general practitioner in Scotstoun, Glasgow and 20 years as an academic GP at the University of Glasgow. Probably, no other member of the university staff, before or since in its 300-year history, had comparable knowledge and experience of the lives and illnesses of nearly 4,000 local people.

Stuart was the first Glasgow GP in modern times to obtain an MD degree by research, studying allergy in general practice. For a randomised controlled trial of stepping down corticosteroid therapy for asthma, he recruited more general practices than any previous research study in the city, without drug company funding. He had many attributes, but what most endeared Stuart to his colleagues was his seriousness about having fun.

Stuart was proud of the university department, his university and city and took pleasure in hosting visitors to all three. As the local organiser for an annual scientific conference of the UK Society of Academic Primary Care, held in Glasgow, he was concerned that visitors to the city would be left on their own in the evening. So, he met 50 of them in the town centre and took them out to dinner.

On the previous evening, he had arranged for 35 heads of department to be bused out to Balamha, picked up by a Loch Lomond cruise boat, wined on the afterdeck, transported across the loch to Luss Pier and decanted for dinner at the Lodge on Loch Lomond; he also arranged for a lone piper (the redoubtable David Hannay, formerly Professor of General Practice at the University of Sheffield) to be playing on the island of Inchcailloch as the boat passed, so that he could be picked up and join the company.

Putting a piper ashore on an uninhabited island in the middle of Loch Lomond so that he could be picked up an hour later is a logistical challenge, but Stuart Wood was equal to the task. As was his habit, he cased the scene beforehand, timed the journeys, found a boatman and had the piper delivered at the right time, in the right place, for transfer to the island. In these and other intrigues, his wife Valerie was the driver and chief assistant. They were a team with talents that could have been turned to many tasks. Bank robbery would not have been beyond them.

For a conference dinner in the University of Glasgow's magnificent Bute Hall, Stuart introduced a technique forever after known as 'The Principal's Friend'. Engaging with the university caterers to ensure their best efforts on the night, Stuart let it slip that a very important guest on the night was 'a close friend of the university principal'. The beauty of the technique was that it was not necessary to specify which friend, nor indeed, which principal.

In those days, before 'team building' and 'strategy days', it was possible to organise days out for the university department. After a couple of hotel-based events, with syndicate rooms and flip charts, we abandoned convention for a simple formula. Stuart was given a budget and asked to arrange something for us collectively that we could not do, or were unlikely to do, individually. To begin with, only the departure and return times were known. There followed a series of imaginative excursions.

Preparation beforehand was Stuart's secret weapon. Numerous deals were made with local hostelries and travel companies, promising unspecified 'future business' if initial experience went well.

A good rule was to cross water early in the day, not only for the calming effect but also to leave evil spirits behind. In this way, we visited Mount Stuart on Bute, the Lake Isle of Menteith and Inchholm Abbey on the Firth of Forth, sailing from South Queensferry under the Forth Railway Bridge to get there. Hiring a cruise boat gave us the freedom of Loch Lomond. On one occasion, after a morning walk round Inchcailloch and lunch on the isle of Inchmurrin, over half of the company went water skiing from Cameron House Hotel.

We cycled round the great Cumbrae, circumnavigated the Bass Rock, walked from Irvine to Troon and from Crail to Anstruther (to see the model fishing boats Professor Hamish Barber had donated to the Scottish Fisheries Museum), climbed the Cobbler and the Whangie, perambulated the McEwan Gardens at Dunoon, explored subterranean tunnels under the Royal Mile and, starting in the Balmoral Hotel, set out to find the best dry martini in Edinburgh. History does not record the outcome of that quest.

The zenith was undoubtedly an awayday to Barcelona. Conceived at a Christmas night out and planned after scouring the Ryanair schedules, we undercut the 24-hour conference rate at the Buchanan Arms, Drymen by £1.50. Most of the party stayed in backpacker accommodation in Barcelona's redlight district. A conference room was booked in a Ramblas hotel, where we spent conscientious daylight hours, exactly as we had done years earlier at similar venues in Scotland, but with Barcelona at our disposal in the evening. Most paid for an extra night. Arriving home, we were exhilarated, and relieved, not to find ourselves on the front page of a tabloid newspaper.

Those days are gone. The concept of an 'awayday' has narrowed but has not been improved. In those carefree days, we often left the west of Scotland without academic general practitioners for 24 hours at a time. No one would dare do that now.

18

Reflection

After the uncertainty of asking 54 colleagues to write for this book, not knowing what their contributions would be and whether or how they would fit together, it has been a relief and a pleasure to see the book develop as a coherent whole with consistent messages and several cross references between topics, places and contributors.

The book may be considered as a *caravanserai* or a stopping place along the way, where travellers meet for rest, company, refueling and the sharing of experiences, intelligence and plans. Some authors have already come a long way; others are setting out. Continuing Andrew Lyon's use of the horizon model (Chapter 2), the departure point for many has been Horizon 1, comprising traditional approaches to health care. The default themes of health care systems around the world are specialization, centralization and privatization, reflecting professional, managerial and business interests (1). The gatekeeping functions of primary care, with and without gates (Section 3.1), are a stabilising force, increasing system efficiency in direct proportion to population coverage. Many countries, as described in the contributions from China, Lebanon and sub-Saharan Africa, are setting out to establish this basic function of primary care (Chapter 13).

At a symposium to celebrate his 80th birthday, Julian Tudor Hart reflected that in almost 40 years of practice, he had never seen a case of parents throwing a baby out with the bath water. Such carelessness happens, but usually when consequences are remote from actions. The recent underfunding of the general practice in the United Kingdom, compared to investments in specialist care, is a case in point, weakening care in the community, increasing pressure on other services, unbalancing the system and exacerbating the problem by threatening GP recruitment and retention.

Maintaining the generalist clinical function in the United Kingdom is now a huge challenge. Changing skill mix will help as nurses, pharmacists and administrative staff take on new roles. Such developments need to be evaluated broadly, not only in terms of what the new roles contribute but also their impact on the generalist clinical function, especially continuity, coordination and coverage. The ultimate yardstick is patient experience.

However, the challenge is not just to maintain the status quo. Neither patients with multimorbidity nor health budgets can afford the fragmentation and inefficiency of overspecialised and over-centralised care. This book embraces that challenge, highlighting the generalist clinical function, the importance of serial encounters, the natural hub function of general practice and the need to strengthen what local health systems can offer, with inclusiveness as a fundamental principle and collegiality as a driving mechanism. The exceptional potential of general practice is being imagined and developed (Horizon 2) but still lies ahead (Horizon 3).

No blueprint or 'logic plan' emerges, only a direction of travel, a huge amount of energy and passion, very similar ideas and values and a willingness to share and learn. Local examples differ in detail but are similar in approach.

Many contributions describe how authors have spent or are spending their own time and energy within local teams. Examples of cluster working have mostly involved small numbers of volunteer practices. These are small beginnings. The task of persuading others has barely begun. Only the work reported from East London (Chapter 10) has involved all practices in an area, working together as a whole system. That example shows not only the power of shared information but also the importance of its cultural underpinning.

The career-long examples are all provided by men, reflecting the profession and society when they started out, but the gender balance is shifting and will continue to shift in the future.

I was glad to be able to call on academic colleagues who had 'stepped outside the academy' to engage and work with GP colleagues. Obtaining research grants and publishing high-quality scientific papers are what Universities expect academic GPs to do, but capturing and building on the experience and views of clinical generalists is important and a task for which academic GPs are suited if they please. In the Deep End Projects, the contribution of academic time, coordination and writing skills has been a crucial ingredient. There are academic spin-offs in terms of the types of research that are then possible (Section 3.4).

A key message for practitioners in the United Kingdom is how fortunate we are with well-paid jobs and working in a system in which it is never necessary to consider what investigations and treatments a patient can afford. Nevertheless, there are lessons to learn from other countries, such as the examples of community practice in Brisbane and Pittsburgh which are ahead of us in terms of integrating medical and psychological care (Sections 9.3 and 9.4).

Conserving and protecting the traditional and stabilising aspects of general practice, sometimes called its Essence, is important but not sufficient. The examples selected and described in this book look outwards, developing practices as the hubs of local health systems, building capacity and strengthening relationships with almost everyone – patients, professional colleagues, other services, local communities, politicians, and so on.

All this can be seen as a necessary reconfiguring of health care and the rebalancing of the roles of generalist and specialist clinicians in order to provide better and more efficient care for patients with multimorbidity. As populations get older and funding becomes tighter, the logic of such change is inarguable. However, the role of health care is not just to respond to the problems and challenges of longevity. It is also a potential instrument of social justice addressing differences in longevity, health and well-being between social groups.

The emphasis in this book is not so much on inequalities in health, which is an abstraction based on comparing data from different groups, as on the practical challenge in deprived areas of increasing the volume, quality and consistency of service provided for patients. Unconditional, personalised continuity of care improves health outcomes. If such care is provided for everyone who needs it, population health can be improved and inequalities narrowed. If health care is not best where it is needed most, inequalities in health will widen. This simple insight is absent from most reports and policies on health inequality.

It follows that while most of the ideas and examples described in the book have widespread relevance and application, they are especially relevant in populations lacking good health, including not only areas of blanket socioeconomic deprivation but also pro rata in areas of pocket deprivation. Reversing the Inverse Care Law is important unfinished business.

Hard-pressed patients, practitioners and practices need time and support in order to move to new ways of working. Deep End Projects show that small amounts of additional resource can re-energise general practices. With extended consultations for selected patients, problems can be reviewed, prioritised and used to develop and drive local arrangements for integrated care. In deprived communities where patients often lack health literacy, agency and confidence, referral links need to be short, quick and familiar. Embedding specialist workers in practice teams improves accessibility, uptake and use. Practices can learn from each other as they address these challenges.

The training opportunities described in South Wales, North Dublin and the Deep End GP Pioneer Scheme show that many general practitioners at the start of their careers are attracted by the challenge of working in deprived areas. They need to be supported and connected as an expanding collegiate force.

Social medicine, diagnosing and treating the ills of society, has a place in general practice, not only in addressing the needs of patients but also by collective action, lobbying on behalf of patients (Section 4.3.4 and 4.3.5). As a result of their frontline position, knowledge and experience, general practitioners are at the crossroads of societal change (2). Without fanfare or fuss, they make a difference, working quietly but steadily with patients and local communities.

John Berger's book, *The Fortunate Man*, is often described as the best account of the work of a general practitioner. He also wrote (3),

> .... in the dark age in which we are living and the new world order, the sharing of pain is one of the essential preconditions for a re-finding of dignity and hope. Much pain is unshareable. But the will to share pain is shareable. And from that inevitably inadequate sharing comes a resistance.

By working with the marginalised, the excluded and the underserved, and by spending time with patients lacking health literacy, confidence and agency, a corner is being turned.

Jan De Maeseneer (Section 9.5) describes how

> A citizen in Ledeberg knows, when he/she is in trouble, that he can go to the community health centre or to the social welfare centre and that he/she will be treated respectfully by skilled, empathetic professional people, giving him/her the feeling that he/she is 'part of society' and that everybody counts.

The challenge is to apply these values not only in individual patient encounters but also throughout health systems, matching rhetoric with generous action. By excluding exclusions and building relationships, inclusive health care is a civilising force in an increasingly dangerous, fragmented and uncertain world.

REFERENCES

1. World Health Report 2008. Primary health care now more than ever. World Health Organization, Geneva, Switzerland, 2008.
2. De Maeseneer J. *Family Medicine and Primary Care at the Crossroads of Societal Change*. Leuven, Belgium: LannooCampus Publishers, 2017.
3. Berger J. *Portraits: John Berger on Artists*, Edited by Overton J. London, UK: Verso, 2015. pp. 335–340.

19

Postscript

19.1 THE VIRTUES OF THE RACE

There are men and classes of men that stand above the common herd: the soldier, the sailor and the shepherd not infrequently; the artist rarely; rarer still the clergyman; the physician almost as a rule. He is the flower (such as it is) of our civilisation, and when that stage of man is done with and only to be marvelled at in history, he will be thought to have shared as little as any in the defects of the period and most notably exhibited the virtues of the race.

Generosity he has, such as is possible to those who practice an art, never to those who drive a trade; discretion tested by a hundred secrets; tact tried in a thousand embarrassments and what are more important, Heraclean cheerfulness and courage, so that he brings air and cheer into the sick room and often enough though not as often as he wishes, brings healing.

Robert Louis Stevenson (1)

Robert Louis Stevenson was a sickly child, born and brought up in Edinburgh's New Town in the mid-nineteenth century. His family, famous as pioneering lighthouse engineers, were well off and able to afford the best doctors or, at least, the best-dressed doctors. He had huge experience as a patient and in later life he wrote down his observations.

His doctors had few effective treatments. After making a diagnosis, what they mostly provided was their presence, as Voltaire put it, 'amusing the patient while Nature took its course'. Stevenson was reflecting not so much on the doctor's role as on the doctors he had seen carrying it out.

Personal qualities are still important, as shown by many contributions to this book, but the doctor's role has changed. Nobody is claiming to be the 'flower of civilization'. More modestly, what is the modern meaning of 'sharing as little as any in the defects of the period and most notably exhibiting the virtues of the race'? This book has tried to answer that question, as it applies to generalist clinicians, responding unconditionally, at least initially, to whatever problem or combination of problems a patient may present.

Diagnosis and treatment in the consultation remain the distinguishing features of medical practice, but in reviewing the past, present and future of what health care can and could achieve, traditional clinical skills are essential but not sufficient.

Since Julian Tudor Hart's pioneering work in the 1960s, 1970s and 1980s, (Section 4.2.2) population medicine, with its implications for practice organisation, information and skill-mix, has become a routine.

Practices are now looking outwards to their communities, establishing links and building capacity to help patients live longer and better in the community, preventing, postponing and lessening the complications of multimorbidity.

Developing long-term productive relationships continues to be the cornerstone of generalist clinical practice, but increasingly the focus is on building similar relationships with professional colleagues, other services and local communities.

With their intrinsic strengths of contact, continuity, coordination, coverage, flexibility and trust, general practices are the natural hubs of local health systems but need GP leadership for the exceptional potential of the hub role to be realised.

Underlying these developments is not only the desire for better, more effective, efficient and equitable health care but also the need to rebuild society as a cooperative endeavour, harnessing strengths and without exclusions. Health care is only one part of society but remains as the most obvious expression of societal values. In helping to build strong patient narratives, strong local systems and equity and consistency across the system as a whole, general practitioners have a central role.

19.2 A PHILOSOPHY OF GENERAL PRACTICE

The most unexpected email I ever received read as follows:

> I am a family medicine specialist from Saudi Arabia. I met you six years ago in a conference in Riyadh. In your presentations, you showed us a picture of a group of stones arranged in a very beautiful manner. Can I get that picture, please?

The picture in question captured an art installation by the British outdoor sculptor Andy Goldsworthy. I chose it as a metaphor for general practice and primary care. Using simple materials, and applying a pattern, with imagination, creativity

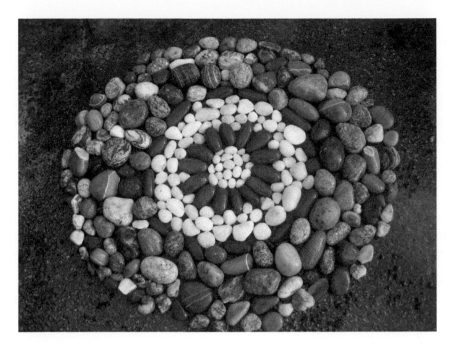

Figure 19.1 Building a pattern.

and purpose, he made something beautiful. Unable to obtain approval to use the original image, I created something similar myself (Figure 19.1).

The French mathematician Poincaré wrote:

> The scientist does not study nature because it is useful to do so. He studies it because he takes pleasure in it because it is beautiful. If something were not beautiful it would not be worth knowing and life would not be worth living. I am not speaking of course of that beauty which strikes the senses, of the beauty of qualities and appearances. I am far from despising this, but it has nothing to do with science. What I mean is that more intimate beauty which comes from the harmonious order of its parts, and which a pure intelligence can grasp ... Intellectual beauty, on the contrary, is self-sufficing and it is for it, more perhaps than the future good of humanity, that the scientist condemns himself to long and painful labours. (1)

Much of science has developed in this way, reducing disease and other phenomena to their component parts, but this is not the way of general practice and primary care. While scientists break things down, practitioners construct. One of the privileges of general practice and family medicine is the opportunity to look after a whole population, whether geographically defined, or a list of people accessing health care at a particular place:

> With great effort any doctor can get to know all his patients, even in a city with a high migrant turnover. Only thus can he learn to think in terms of a responsibility not only of the patient sitting in the surgery, but to the whole population, for whose care he is paid and for whose health he is responsible. He can then see his role as the ultimate custodian of the public health on a defined section of a world front in the war against misery and disease. (2)

The raw material is the consultation. With continuity and coverage, a pattern can be wrought. For individual patients, the serial encounter builds knowledge, experience, confidence and trust, to cope better with life's problems. For the population, audit and the measurement of omission are the keys to equitable care. For the future good of humanity, practitioners take long and painful labours. The effectiveness of primary care depends on the 'harmonious order of its parts'. Primary care is a social construction, made of ordinary materials, mostly men and women, and beautiful in its own way.*

REFERENCES

19.1 The virtues of the race

1. Stevenson RL. *Underwoods*. Chatto & Windus: London, UK, 1912.

19.2 Philosophy of general practice

1. Poincaré H. *Science and Method*. Thoemmes Press: Bristol, UK, 1996.
2. Hart JT. *The Lancet Career Guide for Medical Students*. Lancet Publications: London, UK, 1973.

> It is better to travel hopefully than to arrive and the true success is to labour.
>
> **Robert Louis Stevenson**

---

* Note: This essay is reproduced with permission from the *British Journal of General Practice*. Watt G. Philosophy of general practice: in the eye of the beholder. *Br J Gen Pract* 2014. doi:10.3399/bjgp14 x 682945.

20

Biographies

Attitudes are more important than abilities, motives are more important than methods, character is more important than cleverness and the heart takes precedence over the head. Perseverance is more important than pace. Making the right choices at various junctions in life can be of greater importance than outstanding ability.

Denis P. Burkitt's Advice on Career Building

Behind every contribution in this book, there is a career narrative based on the choices that colleagues made at various stages of their careers. All contributors were invited to describe their careers in 80 words.

Harry Ahmed is a former South Wales GP Academic Fellow and was awarded an NIHR Doctoral Research Fellowship in 2014 to investigate the epidemiology of community-acquired urinary tract infections using routinely collected health record data. He is currently in the final year of his PhD and works part time as a salaried GP in the Rhondda Valleys in South Wales.

Khairat Al Habbal is a family medicine specialist in Beirut and a candidate for an MSc in Global Health Policy from the London School of Hygiene and Tropical Medicine. She is a member of the Alpha Omega Alpha Honor Medical Society and a winner of many awards including the Humanism and Professionalism Award and the Penrose Award. She has a special interest in social medicine, health systems and activism in medicine leading her to teach the former and give workshops on the latter.

Breannon Babbel works for the US National Indian Health Board, which is dedicated to achieving the highest level of health and well-being for American Indians and Alaska Natives. She completed her PhD in Glasgow, Scotland where her research focused on exploring the role of general practice in addressing health inequalities. Originally from Oregon (USA), she received a master of public health and master of public policy degrees from Oregon State University.

Her previous work includes research with the Northwest Portland Area Indian Health Board and Oregon's Marion County Health Department.

David Blane is an academic General Practitioner at the University of Glasgow and has been involved in the Deep End group since 2010, combining clinical work as a part-time GP with teaching and research commitments. He was awarded a master of public health degree with distinction in 2012 and completed his PhD in 2018. He has authored several Deep End reports and manages the group's social media presence. He is an academic coordinator of the Deep End GP Pioneer Scheme.

Megan Blyth graduated from Cardiff University in 2010. After completing her foundation training in South Wales, she travelled to Bundaberg, Australia to work before returning to Cardiff for GP training. She qualified as a general practitioner and was the winner of the RCGP Wales GP Trainee of the year award in 2017. She has an interest in teaching and is currently working as a clinical academic fellow in the South Wales Academic Fellow Scheme.

Kambiz Boomla has been a General Practitioner in Tower Hamlets for 35 years and for many years was the Chair of the Tower Hamlets IT committee helping to establish East London CCGs as among the most digitally mature local health economies in the United Kingdom. He is the Past Chair of the City & East London Local Medical Committee. His R&D interests are in the equitable delivery of digitally enhanced improvement programmes and the governance of information for clinical and third-party uses.

John Budd qualified in 1989 and has been working as a GP since 2001, currently with the Edinburgh Access Practice, caring for people experiencing homelessness. He has worked with the Edinburgh drug problem service and as a rural community doctor in northern KwaZulu-Natal, South Africa, after having completed an MSc in African studies in 1994. Other posts include Chair of the North Edinburgh Drug and Alcohol Centre (NEDAC), steering group member for the Deep End Project and Trustee for the Scottish Drugs Forum.

Peter Cawston qualified in Glasgow in 1993 and after working in France for two years completed GP training and a GP higher professional fellowship in Glasgow, where he has been serving as a Deep End GP since 1999. Other roles have included clinical lecturer, working with several patient groups and leading the Scottish Government's pilot Link Worker Programme. 'The mainstay of my working life, however, has been the long-term relationships with colleagues in my practice team and with our patients on whose trust, forgiveness, good humour and resilience we rely on every day'.

Amanda Connelly has been a GP partner and trainer at Govan Health Centre for 5 years. Prior to this, she worked as a GP partner and trainer in Alexandria, Dunbartonshire for 7.5 years. Her GP training year was enjoyed in her current practice in Govan.

Phil Cotton is the Vice-Chancellor of the University of Rwanda. As an Academic General Practitioner, he was previously the Principal of the College of Medicine and Health Sciences at the University of Rwanda. He continues as a Professor of Learning and Teaching at the University of Glasgow.

Vincent Cubaka is a Medical Doctor with a master's degree in family and community medicine from the University of Rwanda. He holds a PhD in Medicine from Aarhus University. His thesis explored patient–provider communication in primary health care in Rwanda. He practised as a clinician in rural settings for many years. He is currently teaching and researching topics related to primary health care at the University of Rwanda. He is a happy father and husband, and a musician during his spare time.

Jan De Maeseneer chaired the Department of Family Medicine and Primary HealthCare at Ghent University from 1991 to 2017. He contributed to the development of inter-professional Community Health Centres in Belgium, with integrated needs-based capitation financing. His research focused on equity in health, strengthening PHC and improving social accountability. He chaired the European Forum for Primary Care from 2005 to 2017 and was the Secretary-General of The Network: Towards Unity for Health from 2007 to 2015. He chairs the Expert Panel on Effective Ways of Investing in Health, advising the European Commission.

James D. M. Douglas has been a General Practitioner in the Scottish rural town of Fort William since 1979. GP clinical interests include palliative care, learning disability, neurology, mental health and rural health while specialist interests include occupational health and diving medicine. He is an undergraduate and postgraduate GP medical educator and has research publications in occupational asthma, flu diagnosis and flu immunisation. His current research interest is the epidemiology of Lyme disease and its prevention by public health measures. He is the Provost of the North of Scotland Faculty of the RCGP.

Maria Duffy has experience ranging from early childhood in Easterhouse, Glasgow to general practice in Pollok, Glasgow, the intervening years included MB ChB in 1987 (Glasgow), A&E in Australia, psychiatric training scheme, self-constructed GP Training (paediatrics, infectious diseases, geriatrics O&G), medical school teaching, GP appraiser, clinical assistantship in endocrinology, GP educational supervisor, practice lead for the Community Links Project and mother to three (now adult) children. She enjoys the humanity and complexity of general practice and interested in the healing capacity of other human beings.

Bridie Fitzpatrick has 35 years of research experience. This has involved work in a multinational epidemiology project, then health service research concerned with developing and applying new approaches to consult service users and providers, and thereafter designing and managing trials involving complex interventions and vulnerable populations. Her principal interest is in research methodology, and she has gained a reputation for obtaining high recruitment and retention rates as well as high-quality data.

Andrea Fox is a graduate of Sarah Lawrence College, Boston University School of Medicine and the Graduate School of Public Health at the University of Pittsburgh where she is the associate professor in the Department of Family Medicine. She was trained in the social medicine residency program at Montefiore Hospital in the Bronx, where she also completed a fellowship in geriatric medicine. She is the founding medical director of the Squirrel Hill Health Center, a Federally Qualified Health Center dedicated to serving refugees, migrants and other socially excluded people in Pittsburgh.

John Frey qualified in medicine in 1970 from North Western University, Chicago. When he worked with Julian Tudor Hart in South Wales in the early 1970s, he was the first family medicine-trained US doctor to work in the British NHS. He was the head of the Department of Family Medicine at the University of Wisconsin, Madison for 13 years. Although retired, he remains active and is a regular contributor to the BJGP on US health care issues.

John Gillies is from North Uist, Western Isles. He is an Edinburgh graduate and worked in Malawi in the 1980s. He was a rural General Practitioner in Glenluce, then Selkirk for 27 years. He was the Chair of RCGP Scotland from 2010 to 2014 and has published on rural health care, philosophy of medicine and primary health care policy. He co-directs the University of Edinburgh Compassion Initiative, examining compassion in health workplaces. He is the Honorary Professor of General Practice in Edinburgh and Deputy Director of Scottish School of Primary Care.

John Goldie has been a General Practitioner in Easterhouse for 33 years, initially as a registrar then as a partner. During his career, he has witnessed the effects of deprivation on health first hand. He also pursued an interest in medical education and has been a practice trainer, Vocational Studies Tutor and Senior Clinical Tutor at Glasgow University, gaining an MMEd and then an MD. 'This promoted the development of a capacity for reflection, which I have incorporated into my role as a General Practitioner'.

Iona Heath has been a General Practitioner at Kentish Town, London for 35 years. She has written regularly for the *British Medical Journal* and has contributed essays to many other medical journals across the world. She has been particularly interested to explore the nature of general practice, the importance of medical generalism, issues of justice and liberty in relation to health care, the corrosive influence of the medical industrial complex and the commercialisation of medicine, and the challenges posed by disease-mongering, the care of the dying and violence within families.

Sally Hull has been a General Practitioner in Tower Hamlets, East London for 35 years, chairs the Tower Hamlets CCG respiratory programmes and is Clinical Effectiveness Group clinical lead and Local Medical Committee Member. Her R&D interests are in the evaluation of quality improvement programmes in COPD, asthma and renal disease and work on refugees and asylum seekers.

Benjamin Jackson has been a General Practitioner at Conisbrough Group practice, Doncaster, for 15 years, serving some of the most deprived wards in South Yorkshire. An academic interest in GP education led to a period as the Deputy

Director of the Postgraduate School of General Practice, before becoming the Head of GP teaching at Sheffield Medical School. He has been the founder of the Deep End Yorkshire & Humber network and focuses on addressing workforce issues and undergraduate appreciation of the impact of health inequities.

Tracey Johnson is the CEO of Inala Primary Care, a charitable, multidisciplinary, teaching and research active practice in Queensland's most disadvantaged suburban location. In 2015, she undertook a Winston Churchill Memorial Trust Fellowship studying how to bring care out of hospitals and into the community. She is a member of the Evaluation Working Group of the Australian Healthcare Homes Program, the e-mental Health Advisory Committee of the Black Dog Institute and the Primary Care Advisory Group of the Australian Institute of Health and Welfare.

Mark Kelvin has been developing and delivering programmes and services that mitigate the impacts of social injustice for 15 years, whilst also lobbying for and achieving policy change. In 2013, he joined the Health and Social Care Alliance (Scotland) where his main areas of responsibility include the Links Worker Programme, and ALISS, a digital health tool that connects people with their local communities. He is also the Chair of the Board at the social enterprise, Glasgow Watersports.

Andrew Lyon after working in shops and factories, studied sociology and economics at Edinburgh University. After a PhD, he led a community-oriented health programme at Polaroid UK Ltd, before moving to Glasgow to lead the Healthy Cities Programme. He worked for the WHO in Bangladesh and Europe, and then on a Scottish approach to Sustainable Development. With the International Futures Forum, he worked to restore effectiveness in times of rapid change. He chaired the Deep End Steering group from 2009 to 2016.

Becky Macfarlane graduated from Edinburgh in 1993. After registration, she spent a year on an international Christian volunteer team living on a housing estate in East Berlin and two years at Glasgow Bible College with a view to working overseas. She had two salaried GP posts in Glasgow from 2000 to 2017 in practices with large refugee populations. She has helped to coordinate Glasgow Asylum Destitution Action Network since 2010 and currently works mainly in sexual and reproductive health.

Ken McLean retired in 2017 after 37 years as a partner at Carronbank Medical Practice in Denny in Forth Valley. He has had a career-long passion for quality improvement in general practice channelled through the RCGP, which has included chairing the Quality Practice Award and leading on Treating Access and the Effective Interface for RCGP Scotland. He has also sat on both Scottish and UK RCGP Councils and the RCGP Trustee Board.

Stewart Mercer is an academic General Practitioner and has worked clinically in a range of settings including the Deep End. He has been a researcher at Glasgow University for 20 years studying inequalities in health and health care and the importance of empathic, patient-centred care. Since 2008, he has led a programme of research on the needs of patients with multiple complex problems (multimorbidity). He has expertise in the development and evaluation of complex interventions and has been the Director of the Scottish School of Primary Care since 2014.

Brian Milmore graduated from the University of Glasgow in 2006, completing Foundation Training within Glasgow and Ayrshire. Having entered GP training within NHS Ayrshire and Arran, he completed ST3 training in Kilmarnock, subsequently joined Dr Hardie and Partners at Govan Health Centre in 2012 and became a GP Partner in 2013. He is currently the Practice Quality Lead and Clinical Lead for Information in the Govan Social and Health Integration Partnership (SHIP).

John Montgomery has worked in the David Elder Medical Practice, Govan Health Centre since 1987, initially as a registrar, as a partner since 1989 and now as the senior partner. He became a GP trainer, developed an interest in diabetes with the SCI Diabetes Group, had a spell in medical broadcasting with BBC Radio Scotland, was elected as the chair of the South Glasgow GP Committee and now has the Lead Clinician role in the development of the Govan SHIP Project.

Deborah Morrison completed her GP training in 2009, then she continued research and gained her PhD in 2016. She then returned to predominantly clinical work, and alongside GP posts worked with the Glasgow Addictions Services and Youth Health Service. Currently, she works 5 GP sessions per week in a Deep End practice in the east end of Glasgow and 3 GPwSI/research sessions at a Glasgow Diabetes Department. Her current research interests are focussed on vulnerable populations' access to diabetes care.

Anne Mullin has worked in Govan for 24 years as a GP and 'I am exactly where I want to be in my career'. She chairs the Steering Group of General Practitioners at the Deep End.

Austin O'Carroll founded several initiatives addressing health inequities: Safetynet primary care service for over 6,000 marginalised patients annually; GMQ, a primary care service for homeless people; Partnership for Health Equity, a research, education, policy and service delivery collaboration; Curam Healthnet, creating new GP practices in areas of deprivation; and the North Dublin City GP Training programme. He completed a doctorate in ethnographic research into the health service usage behaviours of homeless people. He received the Irish Health Professional of the Year Award in 2015.

Patrick O'Donnell graduated from a rural vocational training scheme in 2012, completed a master's degree in global health and now works as a GP and Clinical Fellow in Social Inclusion at the University of Limerick. He is currently doing a PhD on social exclusion and primary health care. He currently works as a GP in a disadvantaged area of Limerick city and runs clinics for marginalised groups who do not have access to mainstream medical care.

Tom O'Dowd has been a GP in the United Kingdom and Ireland for 40 years, where he has served many roles. Teaching and research informed his work as a regulator and in primary care policy. He has found authenticity in the patient struggle with an illness which is all the more profound where resources are scarce. This has been his motivation in the social entrepreneurship he describes. Being a useful clinician has been central to his career. He is grateful to general practice for a fulfilled life.

Mona Osman is a family medicine specialist at the American University of Beirut and holds Master degrees in public health and business administration. She has 20 years of experience in family medicine, community health, global health, primary health care and health care management. She has worked with non-governmental organizations, academic institutions, private companies, public institutions, international organizations, and United Nation agencies. She founded CHAMPS Fund: The Hicham El Hage Program for Young Hearts and Athletes Health, a humanitarian fund that helps save the lives of young athletes.

Euan Paterson gave medicine not a thought until his higher results, nor general practice until he went to university. He had no idea what general practice would entail, but he admired the style (and sartorial elegance!) of his family's GP in Dunoon. For generalist palliative care, two patients transformed him, though the realisation came much later. As a JHO in 1981: a young man dying of lung cancer. As an inexperienced GP in 1989: a dying retired GP. 'I owe them a huge amount'.

Dominic Patterson has been a GP for 12 years and has an interest in medical education and more particularly how it can be used to help address health inequalities. He founded Fairhealth (fairhealth.org.uk) to further this work and developed the health equity GP curriculum as his master's project. He is a member of the RCGP council and health inequalities standing group.

John Patterson is a General Practitioner and Medical Director of Hope Citadel Healthcare, an NHS Social Enterprise running nine practices covering 31,000 patients in hard-pressed neighbourhoods around Greater Manchester. Their response to the demands of the 'Deep End' was to design a 'Focused Care' model to bias health care access to the most vulnerable and needy households. Three of their practices have been rated 'Outstanding' by CQC. From 2018, he was appointed as the CCO of Oldham CCG.

Tom Ratcliffe is a Modality Partnership General Practitioner with an interest in medical education. He practices in Keighley, West Yorkshire, where he has worked to address health inequity through social prescribing, community engagement and clinical development. In 2015, he helped set up GP at the Deep End Yorkshire and Humber, which is a regional network of GPs operating in socioeconomically deprived areas. He completed his medical degree at the University of Warwick in 2008 and qualified as a GP in 2013.

Douglas Rigg has been a General Practitioner in Keppoch Medical Practice since 2006, during which time the practice has been the 'most deprived' in Scotland. Since 2016, he has been the Cluster Quality Lead GP for the Possilpark and Milton area of Glasgow. Originally from Hong Kong, he studied in Aberdeen before working as a GP trainee across Scotland and in Australia. During his career, he has developed a particular interest regarding health inequalities in cancer care.

Lisa Robins studied medicine at Dundee University. She also completed an intercalated BSc in International Health at Leeds University and graduated in 2009. This was where she first learned about the wider determinants of health. She has an ongoing interest in global health, inequalities in health and marginalised communities. She was trained in Glasgow and has been a GP Pioneer Scheme Fellow at Keppoch Medical Practice since November 2016.

John Robson has been a GP in Tower Hamlets, East London for 37 years, has a long-standing interest in cardiovascular disease, chaired the NICE Guideline 2008 on lipids and CVD risk estimation and was a co-author of the QRisk and QDiabetes scores. He is the CV lead for University College London Partners and Tower Hamlets CCG and Clinical Effectiveness Group lead at QMUL. He has carried out a range of research studies on the evaluation of quality improvement in equitable health service delivery.

Petra Sambale has worked in both the United Kingdom and her native country, Germany. She qualified as a GP in Glasgow and has been a partner in Keppoch Medical Practice since 2000. She values the principles of the NHS and enjoys being a GP trainer in an area of concentrated deprivation. She believes GPs have an important part in addressing health inequalities. Her involvement in the Deep End Steering Group led to her current role as the Lead GP of the Deep End Pioneer Project.

Jamie Sinclair has an MSc in Applied Social Research and is particularly interested in challenging (and changing) hierarchical models of policy and service design, delivery and evaluation. Between 2014 and 2018, he led the Building Connections programme. This body of work informed national and local approaches to collaborative working in Scotland. He recently emigrated to Brisbane, Australia and intends to further develop the methods used during the Building Connections programme.

Susan Smith has worked as a GP in practices in Wales, England and Australia but settled back in Dublin 20 years ago. Her research interests include developing interventions for the equitable primary care of patients with chronic conditions, particularly multimorbidity and related clinical issues such as medicines management. She coordinates the Deep End Ireland Group.

Sanjeev Sridharan is the Director of the Evaluation Centre for Complex Health Interventions at the Li Ka Shing Knowledge Institute at St. Michaels Hospital and Associate Professor at the University of Toronto. Previously, he was the Head of the Evaluation Program at the Research Unit in Health, Behaviour and Change at the University of Edinburgh. He is a former associate editor of the *American*

Journal of Evaluation and is on the boards of the *Canadian Journal of Program Evaluation, New Directions for Evaluation* and the *Journal of Evaluation and Program Planning.*

Kenneth Thompson graduated from Kenyon College, Boston University School of Medicine and the Albert Einstein College of Medicine Psychiatric Residency in the Bronx. He was a postdoctoral fellow in mental health services research at Yale, joined the faculty before going to the University of Pittsburgh. He served as the Medical Director of the Center for Mental Health Services, US Department of Health and Human Services. He is currently the Chief Medical Officer of the Pennsylvania Psychiatric Leadership Council.

Kevin Thompson qualified as a General Practitioner in 1982, was a partner in practice for 32 years and retired in 2014. He was an undergraduate medical student Honorary Lecturer at Cardiff School of Medicine from 1995 to 2014 and a GP Trainer from 2004 to 2014. He has been the Director of the South Wales Academic Fellow Scheme for 12 years.

Elizabeth Walton is a Clinical Lecturer in primary care medicine and a GP in the most deprived area of Sheffield at the Whitehouse Surgery. Her NIHR funding is to develop research and teaching skills with a focus on health inequalities. Her passion to work towards health equity for communities and to support professionals working with vulnerable groups was inspired through witnessing the contrasts in the social determinants of health for patients throughout her career.

Harry Hao-Xiang Wang has been conducting primary care research since 2010 using the Primary Care Assessment Tool in China and started to focus on multimorbidity with a Fellowship awarded under the Hong Kong–Scotland Partners in Postdoctoral Research launched by the Research Grants Council of Hong Kong in collaboration with the UK Scottish Government in 2013. He is now based in Guangzhou and leads population-based cohort studies on long-term conditions and multimorbidity in primary care in Guangdong Province, China.

Graham Watt is an Aberdeen medical graduate and after hospital jobs in Shetland, Leicester, Aberdeen and Nottingham worked as MRC Research Registrar at Glyncorrrwg in South Wales with Julian Tudor Hart. After GP training at Ladywell Medical Centre in Edinburgh and Townhead Health Centre in Glasgow, he completed public health training with posts in epidemiology, health services research management and academic public health. Despite this circuitous route, he had the great good fortune in 1994 to become Norie Miller Professor of General Practice at the University of Glasgow.

Suzanne Williams is Director of Clinical Services and a clinician at Inala Primary Care, a charitable, multidisciplinary, teaching, and research active practice in a disadvantaged area of South East Queensland, Australia. She leads in providing GP management of chronic and complex conditions and is involved in developing team-based care for this group. She has been a provider of general practice-based teaching for registrars for more than 10 years and is currently a supervisor for General Practice Training in Queensland.

Andrea Williamson has been a General Practitioner for 18 years combining clinical practice with marginalised patients, teaching and research at the University of Glasgow. She set up the intercalated degree course 'Global Health in a Primary Care Context' for medical students. She is the deputy chair of the RCGP Health Inequalities Standing Group. What unifies her work is the impact of cumulative adversity over a person's life and what this means for society and how health care should be delivered.

Phil Wilson has been a GP for 30 years, a partner for 24 years in Glasgow and now a sessional GP in Inverness. He worked as a part-time researcher at the University of Glasgow before becoming professor of primary care and rural health at the University of Aberdeen, and he holds visiting professorships at Copenhagen and Glasgow Universities. His researches are focused on the development and evaluation of population-based complex interventions to improve health, particularly the health of children.

In Memoriam: Dr. Julian Tudor Hart (1927–2018)

Julian Tudor Hart died on 1 July 2018, at the age of 91. The following text was read at his funeral, remembering Julian as a doctor.

Julian Tudor Hart always wanted to be a doctor in a mining village, partly because his father had been a colliery doctor in Llanelli; partly it was the romance of mining practice as popularised by AJ Cronin in his book *The Citadel*; but mainly it was the sort of community he wanted to belong to.

And belong he did. As Gerald Davies, a patient, said in the BBC documentary *The Good Doctor*, Julian wasn't aloof, like other doctors, the headmaster and colliery manager. He lived in the village and shared the common experience.

He wrote,

Not one is a stranger; they are not only patients but fellow citizens. From many direct and indirect contacts, for example, in schools, shops and gossip, I have come to understand how ignorant I would be if I knew them only as a doctor seeing them when they were ill.

Julian loved his patients – not romantically, of course. The opposite of love in this context is indifference and Julian was never indifferent. He hated when bad things happened to his patients, especially when they could have been prevented. In his last 28 years at Glyncorrwg, there wasn't a single death in women from cervical cancer.

In his book *A New Kind of Doctor*, he described a 42-year-old man, invalided out of the steel industry after a leg fracture. With no further use for his big muscular body, he had become obese, had high blood pressure and cholesterol, got gout and was drinking too much. Julian described how, after 25 years, 310 consultations and 41 hours of work, initially face to face, eventually side by side, the most satisfying and exciting things had been the events that had not happened: no strokes, no heart attacks, no complications of diabetes. He described this as the real stuff of primary medical care.

At a seminar at the University of Glasgow, we asked Julian what had happened to this patient. Eventually, he had died of something else, a late-onset cancer I think, but when Julian told us this, there was a tear in his eye. His patient had become his friend.

This was Dr 'art', without an 'H', as known to his Glyncorrwg patients. None of this explains why Dr Julian Tudor Hart became famous.

Starting with large numbers of very sick people, huge visiting lists and a working colliery nearby, the Glyncorrwg practice was extremely busy. His initial base was a wooden hut. It took five years to reach a stable position on which he could build.

He became the first doctor in the world to measure the blood pressure of all his patients. Famously, Charlie Dixon was the last man to take part, had the highest blood pressure in the village but was still alive 25 years later. Julian became an international authority on blood pressure control in general practice and wrote a book about it which went to three editions and was translated into several languages, with a companion book for patients.

What he did for patients with high blood pressure, he did for other patients, delivering unconditional, personalised continuity of care. After 25 years he showed that premature mortality was almost 30% lower than in a neighbouring village – the only evidence in the world literature of what a general practitioner can achieve in a lifetime of practice.

Julian didn't do this on his own. When Deborah Perkin was planning her BBC documentary, *The Good Doctor*, I said to her, there is something you have to understand. There's two of them. Mary was his partner and anchor every step of the way.

Glyncorrwg was the first general practice in the UK to receive research funding from the Medical Research Council. Both Mary and Julian had worked with Archie Cochrane and his team at the MRC Epidemiology Unit, where they learned a democratic type of research in which everyone's contribution was important, and the picture wasn't complete until everyone had taken part. And so, there was the Shit Study, the Pee Study, the Salt Studies and the Rat Poison Study, all with astonishing high response rates.

Scientific knowledge was a guiding light, which Julian both used and produced. He counted as scientists anyone who measured, or audited, what they did and was honest with the results. Brecht's The Life of Galileo was his favourite play and he often quoted Brecht's line, 'The figures compel us'. Julian didn't pursue knowledge for its own sake. His research always had the direct purpose of helping to improve people's lives.

He spoke and wrote widely with a talent for the telling phrase. His Inverse Care Law stated that the availability of good medical care tends to vary inversely with the need for it in the population served, or as he put it more simply, 'People without shoes are clearly the ones who need shoes the most'.

Increased dental charges would give a financial incentive to patients to look after their "teeth"', said Sir Keith Joseph, a Conservative Secretary for

Social Services. Julian commented, 'The government has not yet raised the tax on coffins to reduce mortality, but Sir Keith is assured of a place in the history of preventive medicine'.

Julian's friend and fellow GP, John Coope from Bollington in Lancashire, commented that one of Julian's talents was his nose for what mattered in the published literature. In his book *The Political Economy of Health*, that magpie tendency was on display, the footnotes alone comprising one-third of the book and worth reading on their own. A Google search could never assemble such a mix. Goodness knows what readers made of it in the Chinese translation.

He had invitations to lecture all over the world – the United States, Australia, Kazakhstan, Italy, Spain in particular. Julian could do the formal lecture but for brilliance and exhilarating an audience he was best in impromptu, unscripted exchange.

When principles were at stake, Julian could and often did argue until the cows came home. In his younger years he took no prisoners. A famous medical professor, internationally renowned, reflected that he had been called many things, but never a snail.

A well-known TV doctor arrived in the village to interview Julian for her TV programme, determined to cast him in the role of a doctor who made life or death decisions concerning his patients' access to renal dialysis and transplant. They battled for a whole afternoon, she trying to get Julian to say things that fitted her script. He defied her, ending every sentence by mentioning how much dialysis and transplant surgery the cost of a single Trident missile could buy. She went away defeated and empty-handed.

I was surprised once at Paddington Station to see him with a copy of the London Times. He was no fan of the Murdoch press. On boarding the 125 for South Wales, he laid out the newspaper as a tablecloth and spread out a messy, aromatic Indian carry-out meal. If businessmen in their suits wanted to sit near us, they were very welcome.

Standing for election to the Council of the Royal College of General Practitioners, Julian topped the poll. What he offered GPs was an image of themselves as credible and important members of the medical profession, alongside specialists, not beneath them.

Julian was humble in himself but ambitious for his ideas. He accepted with ambivalence the honours and sentimental treatment that came with age but never lost his edge, and if we are to celebrate his life it should be by holding to the principles he held dear.

The work of a general practitioner is immeasurably enhanced by working in, with and for a local community, for long enough to make a difference.

Everyone is important, the last person as important as the first, and the work isn't done until everyone is onboard.

Julian embodied the 'worried doctor', seeing it as his job to anticipate patients' problems, not wait for them to happen, and to avoid them by joint endeavour.

Drawing on Marx, he saw health care as a form of production, producing not profits but social value, achieved not by the doctor alone but by doctors and patients together, transferring knowledge, building confidence, initially face to face, eventually side by side.

The NHS is not a business but a social institution based on mutuality and trust – the ultimate gift economy, getting what you need, giving what you can, like blood transfusion writ large, a model for how society might run as a whole. In rebuilding society, cooperation would trump competition, not marginally, but as steam once surpassed horsepower. The Glyncorrwg research studies showed glimpses of that social power.

Julian's gift to us today is not the example of how he worked out these values in the microcosm of a Welsh mining village over 25 years ago; it is the challenge of how we adopt, promote and give practical expression to his values in local communities in the future. In honouring his memory, there is work to do.

Graham Watt

Index

Note: Page numbers in italic and bold refer to figures and tables, respectively.